Famous People Don't Get Fat

Here are the secrets
you need to keep you
as slim as the stars

Famous People Don't Get Fat

Adele Parker

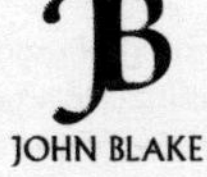

Published By John Blake Publishing Ltd,
3 Bramber Court, 2 Bramber Road,
London W14 9PB, England

www.blake.co.uk

First published in paperback in 2008

ISBN 978 1 84454 494 3

British Library Cataloguing-in-Publication date:

A catalogue record for this book is available from the British Library.

Design by www.envydesign.co.uk

Printed and bound in Great Britain by CPI Bookmarque, Croydon CR0 4TD

3 5 7 9 10 8 6 4 2

Papers used by John Blake Publishing are natural, recyclable products made from wood grown in sustainable forests. The manufacturing processes conform to the environmental regulations of the country of origin.

Every attempt has been made to contact the relevant copyright-holders, but some were unavailable. We would be grateful if the appropriate people could contact us.

The publishers would like to make it clear that this book is not authorised or endorsed by any of the celebrities featured within.

The information contained in this publication is in no way to be considered a substitute with a competent health care professional. Skilled medical opinion is advised on specific health complaints.

Contents

Introduction

CELEBRITIES! Love 'em or loathe 'em, nowadays we don't seem to be able to get enough of them. Every time we open a newspaper or turn on the TV, we are assaulted with a barrage of celebrity news and gossip to keep even the most ardent celeb-watcher satisfied.

If you're a celebrity, of course, fame is what you need to keep your career on the move. The moment you lose that essential coverage is the moment the public starts to forget about you, so the career-minded celebrity has to make sure at all costs that he or she is on the front page as often as is humanly possible.

And to do this they have to look fantastic. For this

reason alone, it's hardly surprising that the celebrities we know and love have come up with all sorts of weird and wonderful ways of losing weight. For them, staying slim is a religion, and they know that in the fickle world of stardom the moment they cease to be able to slip into that little Versace number for that A-list opening night could be the start of the slippery slope down to – horror of horrors – obscurity! Do you fancy living like that? I'm not sure I do...

But that doesn't mean to say that the enthusiastic slimmer can't learn a great deal from a little light star-gazing. These people do, after all, devote a great deal of time and money into keeping their figures just the way their adoring public likes them. And while the wallet-busting accumulation of personal trainers, personal dieticians and personal chefs may be beyond the reach of you and me, it doesn't mean we can't keep an eye on our favourite actresses, pop stars and TV presenters and maybe appropriate a few of their techniques for ourselves.

That's what this book is all about. In the pages that follow you'll find hints, tips, diet plans, recipes – all the weird and wonderful ways the famous become slim and stay that way. Some of them are obvious; some might seem a little wacky, but what I have tried to do is pick the most sensible, effective and healthy slimming secrets of the rich and famous.

We can all think of a celebrity or two who seems at some stage to have taken things a bit too far. Sometimes their slimming secrets can be downright cranky, and instead of looking lithe and vibrant they end up looking skeletal and unhealthy. I'm not interested in those sorts of slimming secrets, and neither should you be. The many weight-loss programmes in this book have been selected and designed to be safe, effective and good for you.

So go ahead: experiment with the different methods of weight loss described here until you find which star's slimming secrets are right for you. They may not win you an Oscar, but they should lead to you being slimmer, more confident and more at ease with your own body. And that's what successful dieting is all about, isn't it?

CONVERSION TABLES

LIQUID MEASURES			
Fluid Ounces	American	British (*Imperial*)	Millilitres
	1 teaspoon	1 teaspoon	5
¼	2 teaspoons	1 dessertspoon	10
½	1 tablespoon	1 tablespoon	14
1	2 tablespoons	2 tablespoons	28
2	¼ cup	4 tablespoons	56
4	½ cup		110
5		¼ pint	140
6	¾ cup		170
8	1 cup		225
9			250
10	1¼ cups	½ pint	280
12	1½ cups		340
15		¾ pint	420
16	2 cups		450
18	2 ¼ cups		500
20	2 ½ cups	1 pint	560
24	3 cups		675
25		1 ¼ pints	700
27	3 ½ cups		750
30	3 ¾ cups	1½ pints	840
32	4 cups or 1 quart		900
35		1¾ pints	980
36	4 ½ cups		1000 (1L)
40	5 cups	2 pints	1120

SOLID MEASURES			
Imperial		Metric	
Ounces	Pounds	Grams	Kilos
1		28	
2		56	
3½		100	
4	¼	112	
5		140	
6		168	
8	½	225	
9		250	¼
12	¾	340	
16	1	450	
18		500	½
20	1¼	560	
24	1½	675	
27		750	¾
28	1¾	780	
32	2	900	
36	2¼	1000	1

OVEN TEMPERATURES		
Fahrenheit	Celsius	Gas Mark
225	110	¼
250	130	½
275	140	1
300	150	2
325	170	3
350	180	4
375	190	5
400	200	6
425	220	7
450	230	8
475	240	9

Kirstie Alley

THE BEAUTIFUL Kirstie Alley certainly lit up our screens when she starred in the hit TV series *Cheers*. And she's managed to keep those curves that made Ted Danson drool as she's grown older and her successful acting career has moved on. But nobody's perfect, and her occasionally fluctuating weight has been the subject of attention for some years now. When the chips are down, though, she always manages to look fantastic. How does she do it?

When she really needs to lose weight fast, Kirstie will cut out food for up to two whole days, and drink nothing but herbal teas. Sounds crazy? Well, it's not something you should do too often, but as long as you are sensible it can be a fantastic way of slimming down for a special occasion – or an important day's filming if you're a top actress! What's more, herbal teas and infusions can have some extremely beneficial effects. Here are some suggestions:

Chamomile

Chamomile tea is very good for the digestion and for easing stomach cramps. It can help soothe menstrual pain, and is well known for helping you to relax and sleep. You can even use it externally on bruises and burns by dabbing a cool chamomile teabag on to your skin.

Lemon Balm

Lemon Balm tea is a well-known remedy for battling the onset of low spirits, while at the same time it's good for those who want to relax. It is also thought to prevent colds.

Raspberry Leaf

Raspberry Leaf tea is a veritable potion of vitamins and minerals, providing you with A, B+, C and E vitamins, as well as calcium, iron and magnesium. For this reason alone it is excellent if you are following a detox regime. It is also very good for pregnant women and new mothers: it can reduce morning sickness and helps the production of breast milk.

Peppermint

Peppermint tea is wonderful for treating indigestion, but that's not where its usefulness ends. It is high in B vitamins, the fumes are excellent for relieving a blocked nose and it can help prevent gallstones.

So, as you can see, there are many other reasons for doing as Kirstie Alley does and detoxing on herbal teas.

For a more long-term slimming regime, Kirstie, like many other celebrities, follows a high-protein, low-carbohydrate slimming regime (see page 331 for more on these).

Coleen McLoughlin avoids the temptation of ordering in calorie-laden takeaways by making healthier options such as home-made, low-fat versions of her favourite treats.

Jennifer Aniston

SHE'S BEEN married to Brad Pitt, and she's starred in the biggest TV show in the world. You don't get all this without a celebrity body to die for! And Jennifer Aniston sure has that. But how does she maintain it?

High-protein, low-carbohydrate diets are all the rage in Hollywood. All sorts of stars, including Matt LeBlanc, Madonna, Sarah Jessica Parker, Matthew Perry and Winona Ryder, are said to be big fans. Jennifer Aniston reckons on consuming a ratio of 40 per cent carbohydrate, 30 per cent protein and 30 per cent fat in order to maintain her slinky figure, and if you try the following recipes which stick to this ratio, you might well find yourself losing weight like Jennifer. She is reported as saying, 'It was amazing to see this other body emerge. I never knew I had it in me.' Perhaps you never knew you had it in you either...

Don't try this for more than a month to begin with; and if you want to research high-protein diets in more detail, the most widely followed one is the Zone Diet, devised by Dr Barry Sears. The Atkins Diet, devised by Dr Robert Atkins, is a stricter version. (See page 332 for more on these diets.)

DAY 1

BREAKFAST

240ml low-fat cottage cheese

1 Granny Smith apple, cored and chopped

6 peanuts, chopped

1 kiwi fruit

1 tangerine

Mix the apple and peanuts with the cheese and surround with the sliced kiwi and the segmented tangerine.

LUNCH

Peruvian Ceviche

(Serves 4)

160g very fresh white fish fillets

½ medium onion, chopped

½ orange

1 lime

½ tablespoon fresh marjoram, chopped

½ tablespoon fresh coriander, chopped

1 ¼ teaspoons virgin olive oil

a pinch of Stevia sweetener (available from health food shops)

a splash of Tabasco sauce

115g radishes, sliced

1 large lettuce heart

salt and freshly ground black pepper

Skin the fish and cut into small pieces. Add the onion to the fish. Pour the juice of the orange and the limes over the fish and onion. Cover and refrigerate, if possible overnight but for at least 6 hours, until the fish is opaque.

Add the herbs to the fish, along with the olive oil and the Tabasco sauce. Season to taste and mix thoroughly. Keep in a cool place for about 1 hour, allowing the flavours to develop.

Shred the lettuce and divide between 4 plates. Pile the fish on the top and garnish with the lime wedges and radishes.

DINNER

Veal and Mushrooms with Vegetables and a Tomato Coulis

(Serves 2)

125g veal

1½ teaspoon virgin olive oil

125g mushrooms

4 spring onions, finely chopped

2 tomatoes, chopped, skinned and seeded

150ml vegetable stock

1 bay leaf

170g spinach

115g cauliflower

Cut the veal into strips and sauté quickly in half the oil. Remove from pan, add the sliced mushrooms and cook until brown. Mix with the veal. Keep warm.

Sauté the spring onions with the remainder of the oil until they are soft. Add the tomatoes and cook until soft. Add the stock and the bay leaf and simmer gently for a few minutes to make a sauce.

Wilt the spinach and steam the cauliflower.

Pour the sauce over the veal and mushrooms and serve with the spinach and cauliflower.

DESSERT

70g mandarins

Angelina Jolie staves off those hunger pangs by snacking on low-fat breakfast cereals. Her favourites are Cheerios – she calls them 'the greatest food in the world'.

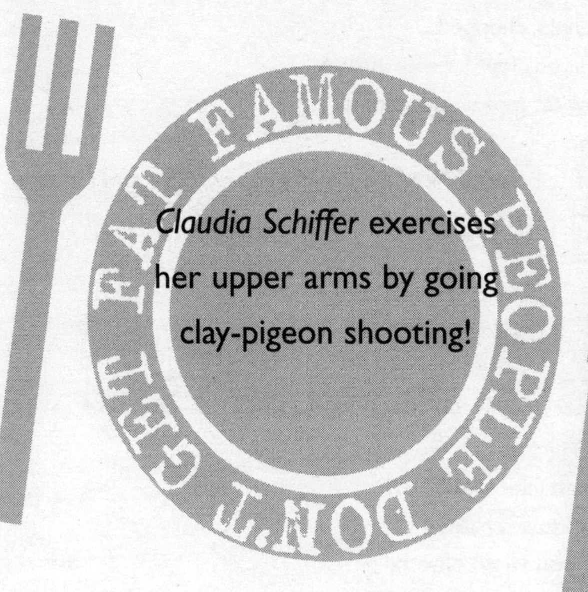

Claudia Schiffer exercises her upper arms by going clay-pigeon shooting!

DAY 2

BREAKFAST

2 slices wholegrain bread

60g chicken breast, cooked and chopped

1 stick celery, chopped

12 peanuts, chopped

2 teaspoons low-fat mayonnaise

60g low-fat mozzarella cheese

Toast the bread. Combine the chicken, celery and peanuts with the mayonnaise and serve on the toast with the mozzarella.

LUNCH

Steak and Hot Bean Salad

(Serves 1)

125g lean fillet steak

1 garlic clove, crushed

1 teaspoon virgin olive oil

½ small lemon

2 small grilled tomatoes

Salad of 4 chopped spring onions, 170g salad spinach, 85g green beans and 225g uncooked chopped mushrooms, salt and freshly ground black pepper.

Spread the garlic on the steak and spray with a little oil. Grill with the tomatoes. Combine the oil and lemon juice and flavour with a little mustard and salt and pepper. Toss the spinach, spring onions and mushrooms together. Lightly cook the beans and serve hot on the salad.

Dish the steak and tomatoes and serve the salad on the side.

DINNER

Tuna and Rice Salad

(Serves 1)

115g canned tuna in spring water
1 teaspoon virgin olive oil
1 red onion, chopped
50g brown rice
juice of ½ lemon
55g frozen peas
1 tomato, cut into sections
1–2 parsley sprigs

Sauté the onion in the oil until soft. Add the rice and mix well. Cook the rice according to the instructions on the packet until all the liquid has evaporated. Cook the peas and mix with the rice, lemon juice and tuna.

Garnish with the tomato and parsley.

DAY 3

BREAKFAST

30g oats

240ml skimmed milk

60ml low-fat cottage cheese

4 spring onions

60g lean ham

100g pineapple, chopped

1 apple, chopped

1 tablespoon chives, chopped

Pour the milk over the oats and serve.

Cut the ham into strips, combine with the pineapple, apple and cheese and serve sprinkled with the chives.

Lamb and Vegetable Hotpot

(Serves 1)

115g lean lamb, cut into mouth-sized pieces
1 medium onion, chopped
1 garlic clove, crushed
30g carrots, diced
85g mushrooms, sliced
85g Chinese cabbage, shredded
2 tomatoes, skinned, seeded and chopped
2 teaspoons cornflour
1½ teaspoons virgin olive oil
1 tablespoon Worcestershire sauce
juice of ½ lemon
parsley, chopped

Heat the oil in a non-stick wok and sauté the onions, garlic and carrots until they have softened a little. Add the lamb and cook until brown. Add the mushrooms and cabbage and stir-fry until cooked.

Mix the cornflour with 75ml of water, the Worcestershire sauce and the lemon juice, and thicken the mixture. Add the tomatoes to warm through. Serve sprinkled with the parsley.

DINNER

Vegetable Medley with Tofu

(Serves 1)

30g firm tofu, diced

2 tomatoes, skinned, seeded and chopped

1 large red pepper

1 large yellow pepper

85g leeks, diced

4 sticks celery, trimmed and diced

1 onion, chopped

1 teaspoon virgin olive oil

1 garlic clove, crushed

1 teaspoon Worcestershire sauce

1 tablespoon white wine vinegar

juice and zest of ½ lemon

2 teaspoons cornflour

Add a little of the oil to a non-stick pan and when hot add the tofu and the Worcestershire sauce and cook until the tofu is nice and brown. Add the remaining oil to another pan and cook all the vegetables except the tomatoes until they are tender.

Mix the cornflour with 90ml of water and add to the pan, together with the lemon juice and zest, and bring to a simmer. Add the tomatoes and fold in the tofu.

DAY 4

BREAKFAST

(Serves 1)

175ml low-fat cottage cheese flavoured with ground cinnamon to taste
½ grapefruit, segmented
115g fruit cocktail in juice (drained)
1 nectarine, sliced
4 teaspoons flaked almonds, toasted

Combine the cheese and the fruit and sprinkle with the nuts.

LUNCH

Chicken and Prawn Salad

(Serves 1)

30g skinless chicken breast, diced
130g prawns
225g lettuce, shredded
½ grapefruit, segmented
8 spring onions, chopped
40g canned red kidney beans, well rinsed
40g canned chickpeas, well rinsed
1 teaspoon virgin olive oil
60ml chicken stock
½ tablespoon balsamic vinegar
1 tablespoon fresh basil, shredded
juice of ½ lemon

Heat ½ teaspoon of the oil in a non-stick wok. Sprinkle the chicken and prawns with the lemon juice and cook them over a medium heat for about 4 minutes.

Mix the vinegar, stock and basil in a small bowl.

Combine the remainder of the ingredients in a salad bowl, top with the chicken and prawns and pour over the dressing.

DINNER

Sweet and Sour Tenderloin

(Serves 1)

115g pork tenderloin sliced into medallions
1½ apples, diced
1 little gem lettuce, sliced
½ tablespoon honey
1 small red onion, chopped
2 small apricots, chopped
1 teaspoon virgin olive oil
½ teaspoon soy sauce
1 tablespoon water flavoured with a squeeze of lime
2 teaspoons fresh sage, chopped
2 teaspoons grained mustard
1 tablespoon white wine vinegar
2 tablespoons red wine vinegar
salt and freshly ground black pepper

Combine half the oil, the mustard, the white wine vinegar and half the honey. Add the pork and coat the meat well. Cover and leave to marinate for about 1 hour.

Sauté the meat in a non-stick pan until it is cooked through. Stir in the apples, apricots, the remainder of the honey, the sage and the lime water.

Mix together the remaining oil, the soy sauce, the red wine vinegar and the salt and pepper. Toss the lettuce and onion in this mixture and top with the pork and fruit.

DAY 5

BREAKFAST

Ham and Vegetable Breakfast

(Serves 1)

75g lean ham

2 medium tomatoes, skinned, seeded and chopped

4 spring onions, chopped

125g chestnut mushrooms, sliced

2 sticks celery, chopped

75g asparagus spears

1 teaspoon virgin olive oil

1 garlic cloves, crushed

a few drops of Tabasco sauce

1 tablespoon cider vinegar

2 teaspoons parsley, chopped

salt and freshly ground black pepper

Heat the oil in a non-stick pan. Combine the vegetables with the garlic, Tabasco sauce, cider vinegar, parsley, salt and pepper, and sauté for 6 minutes until just tender. Add the ham and cook for 2 minutes.

LUNCH

Oriental Stir-fry

(Serves 1)

115g lean fillet steak, diced

85g Chinese cabbage, shredded

75g shitake mushrooms, sliced

75g mangetout, sliced

2 teaspoons cornflour

2 tomatoes, skinned and seeded

2 red onions, chopped

1 teaspoon virgin olive oil

2 tablespoons balsamic vinegar

1 garlic clove, crushed

½ teaspoon dried mixed herbs

½ teaspoon Tabasco sauce (or to taste)

juice of ½ lemon

Heat the oil in a large non-stick pan or wok and sauté the beef until golden brown. Deglaze the pan with the vinegar, Tabasco sauce, water and lemon juice. Add all the ingredients except the tomato, cornflour and herbs and cook until tender. Stir in the tomatoes and cornflour (mixed with 3 tablespoons of water) and cook, while stirring, for 4 minutes, until the tomatoes are heated through and the mixture thickens. Sprinkle with the mixed herbs.

DINNER

Lamb and Vegetable Casserole

(Serves 1)

85g lean lamb, diced

170g leeks, chopped

85g Swiss chard, torn

½ apple, chopped

40g canned chickpeas (drained and rinsed)

1 teaspoon virgin olive oil

½ teaspoon mixed spice

good pinch cayenne pepper

juice of ½ lemon

salt and freshly ground black pepper

Heat the oil in a pan and sauté the lamb and leeks until lightly browned. Add 120ml of water, flavoured with the lemon juice, mixed spice, cayenne and salt and pepper to taste. Cover, reduce the heat and simmer for 10 minutes. Add the Swiss chard, apple and chickpeas. Bring to the boil and simmer for 2 minutes to heat through. Place the lamb on a dish and use a slotted spoon to spread the vegetables around it.

DAY 6

BREAKFAST

Stuffed Pears

(Serves 1)

170ml low-fat cottage cheese

120ml natural low-fat yogurt

1 pear, cored and halved lengthwise (dip in lemon juice to avoid discolouring)

2 prunes, stoned and diced

4 teaspoons flaked almonds

¼ teaspoon ground mace

½ teaspoon lemon zest

¼ teaspoon ground cardamom

Spoon the prunes into the pear halves. Cook in a microwave for 4 minutes on high setting.

Combine the yogurt, mace, lemon zest and cardamom.

Place the cottage cheese on a plate and sprinkle with the almonds. When the pear halves are quite soft, lay them on the cheese, top with the yogurt and serve.

Seafood Sauté

(Serves 1)

60g raw medium prawns, shelled, de-veined and cut into large dices
60g scallops, cut into large dices
240ml semi-skimmed milk
85g leek, diced
40g water chestnuts, diced
2 tomatoes, skinned, seeded and chopped
1 teaspoon virgin olive oil
240ml chicken stock
1 garlic clove, crushed
2 tablespoons fresh coriander, chopped
1 teaspoon celery seeds
½ teaspoon Tabasco sauce

Heat a non-stick pan, add oil and sauté the leeks, water chestnuts, coriander, Tabasco sauce and celery seeds until tender. Add the prawns, scallops and garlic. Cook for 4 minutes until the prawns are pink and the scallops are opaque. Add the tomatoes and chicken stock. Simmer for about 5 minutes. Add the milk and simmer for a further 3 minutes. Mix the cornflour with a little water or white wine and stir until the stock thickens.

DINNER

Chicken Curry with Chinese Cabbage

(Serves 1)

115g skinless chicken breast, diced
120ml salsa (according to taste)
1 red onion, chopped
40g cannellini beans
40g black beans
85g cabbage, shredded
2 garlic cloves, crushed
2 teaspoons curry powder
salt and freshly ground black pepper

Heat a non-stick pan and add the oil. Sauté the chicken until it is slightly brown, then add the garlic and continue cooking gently until the chicken is cooked through. Add the salsa, onion, cannellini beans, black beans, curry powder, and salt and pepper to taste.

Spray a wok with oil and stir-fry the cabbage until cooked but still crisp.

Dish the cabbage and top with the chicken and vegetables.

DAY 7

BREAKFAST

1-egg omelette made with 1 teaspoon of virgin olive oil and filled with 8 chopped spring onions, 2 tomatoes, skinned, seeded and chopped. When cooked, sprinkle with 30g low-fat grated cheese and grill for a few seconds. Serve with 60g heated baked beans.

LUNCH

Mixed Salad with Sole Fillet

(Serves 2)

170g fillet of sole
255g lettuce
130g bean sprouts
1 large red pepper, cut into strips
1 large green pepper, cut into strips
35g carrots, grated
120g grapes, seeded
1 teaspoon virgin olive oil
2 teaspoons fresh lemon juice
2 tablespoons fresh basil, shredded

Spray a non-stick pan with oil and sauté the sole for 2–3 minutes. Combine the lettuce, bean sprouts, peppers, carrots and grapes in a bowl. Whisk the oil and lemon juice together and toss into the salad. Top with the fish and sprinkle with the basil.

DINNER

Turkey Sauté with Vegetable and Fruit

(Serves 1)

115g skinless turkey breast, cut into strips
85g leeks, finely chopped
170g chestnut mushrooms, sliced
120ml unsweetened apple purée
2 teaspoons cornflour
1 teaspoon virgin olive oil
2 teaspoons white wine vinegar
juice of ½ small orange
1 teaspoon dill, freshly chopped
juice of ½ lemon

Sauté the turkey and leeks in half the oil in a non-stick pan. Remove from pan and keep warm. Add the remaining oil and sauté the mushrooms for about 4 minutes. Mix the cornflour with 250ml of water, add all the remaining ingredients and cook until thickened. Spoon on to serving plate and top with the turkey.

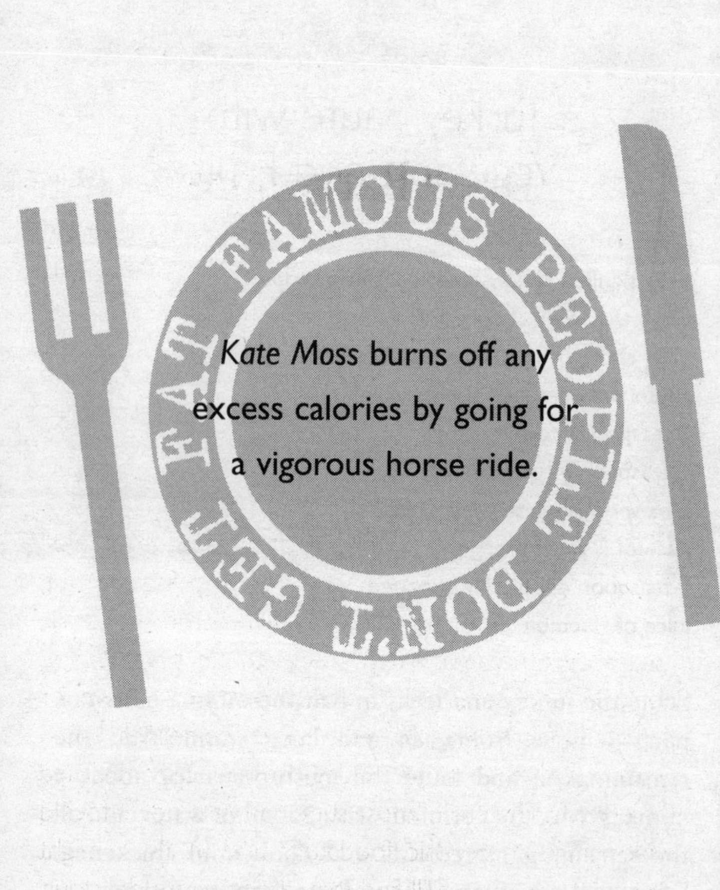
FAMOUS PEOPLE DON'T GET FAT
Kate Moss burns off any excess calories by going for a vigorous horse ride.

Drew Barrymore

SEXY DREW Barrymore follows an organic vegan diet. So what does that mean? Well, meat and fish are out, but so are all other animal products – so no eggs, milk, cream or other dairy items. And to be organic, you need to choose products that have been grown or produced according to very strict guidelines – no artificial additives, no pesticides or genetically modified ingredients. Thankfully, most supermarkets now stock a wide range of organic foodstuffs and, while it might cost a little extra, you'll find that it is far more delicious, better for you and better for the planet!

Following a vegan diet might seem at first to be a little restrictive, but there is no reason why you shouldn't eat just as well on this regime as on any other. Here are a few recipe suggestions to get you started:

Chickpea and Vegetable Combo

(Serves 2–4)

1 can chickpeas
1 garlic clove, roughly chopped
juice of ½ lemon
a little olive oil
a few baby carrots
1 courgette, cut into batons
4 thick slices aubergine
salt and freshly ground black pepper

Drain the chickpeas and keep about half the liquid. Blend in a liquidiser with the liquid you have kept from the can, the lemon juice, the garlic, the seasoning and just a splash of olive oil to moisten the mixture.

Brush the vegetables with a very little olive oil and place on a hot griddle. Cook, turning frequently, until soft and golden. Serve with the chickpea mixture.

Orange and Fennel Salad

(Serves 4)
4 juicy oranges, peeled and segmented
2 small red onions, peeled and finely sliced
1 bulb of fennel, peeled and finely sliced
juice of 1 lime
a small amount of olive oil
salt and freshly ground black pepper

Combine all the ingredients with the olive oil and serve.

Perfect Tomato Soup

(Serves 4)
900g ripe tomatoes, skinned and diced
1 tablespoon olive oil
1 large onion, finely sliced
2 large garlic cloves, crushed
1 tablespoon lemon juice
a little sweetener
salt and freshly ground black pepper

Heat the oil in a large saucepan, add the onions and garlic and cook until soft but not brown. Add the tomatoes, cook for 10–15 minutes, then add the lemon juice, a pinch of sweetener and 350ml of water. Bring to the boil, then simmer very gently for about 10 minutes. Liquidise, reheat if necessary, season and serve.

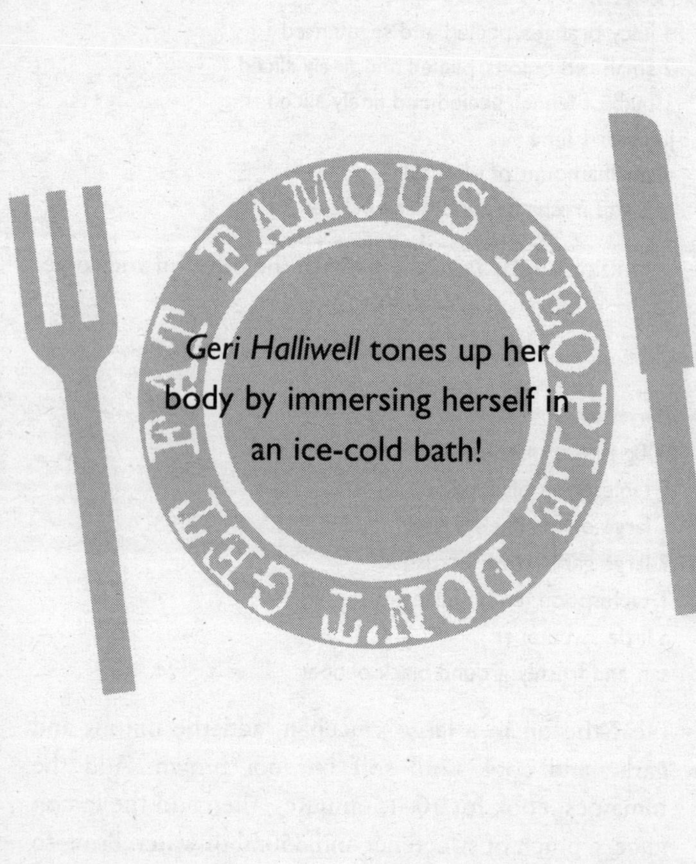
FAMOUS PEOPLE DON'T GET FAT
Geri Halliwell tones up her body by immersing herself in an ice-cold bath!

Sophie Dahl keeps in trim by climbing the stairs to her third-floor apartment instead of taking the elevator. She also regularly drinks cups of green tea, which is thought to speed up the metabolism and reduce cholesterol levels.

Wild Rice Salad

(Serves 4)

250g wild rice

4 sticks celery, finely chopped

1 red pepper, deseeded and finely diced

2 cooked beetroot, roughly diced

a small bunch of spring onions, finely chopped

a small bunch of flat leaf parsley, finely chopped

low-calorie French dressing to moisten

Cook the rice according to the instructions on the packet, then allow to cool. Combine all the remaining ingredients with the rice and serve.

Peppered Strawberries

Sprinkle some ripe strawberries with some freshly squeezed orange juice, sprinkle with pepper and serve. An odd-sounding combination, but a delicious one.

Victoria Beckham

VICTORIA BECKHAM is the queen of slim – not bad for a woman who's had three babies. But the pounds haven't just fallen off her, especially as she admitted to being addicted to fatty foods during her third pregnancy with Cruz. Fortunately for Posh, she was living in Spain at the time. At the advice of her Spanish doctors, she regained her enviable post-pregnancy figure by following an ordinary Spanish diet – no hardship for her, as she is known to love the paella, olives and omelettes of Spanish cuisine; and good news for food-lovers as it is hearty as well as healthy. The benefits of the Mediterranean diet are well known, so it's hardly surprising that Victoria reverted to her A-list physique in no time at all.

What follows is a five-day healthy Spanish eating regime of the type Victoria liked so much (with some meatier dishes for David and the boys) – delicious, authentic and, like Victoria herself, with a touch of class. Let's just hope that now she's moved to LA, she manages to keep away from those all-American burgers!

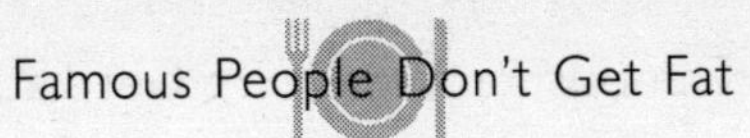

DAY 1

BREAKFAST

2 slices chilled fresh melon sprinkled with lime juice

Small portion Spanish Tortilla served with sliced fresh tomato

LUNCH

Gazpacho with crisp bread rolls

DINNER

Cauliflower Salad Niçoise

Chuletas (Spanish Steaks)

Higos Borrachos (Brandied figs)

DAY 2

BREAKFAST

Fresh grapefruit

Revelto con Setas (eggs with mushrooms)

LUNCH

Baked Fish Spanish style

Large green salad dressed with lemon juice

Bread rolls

DINNER

Paella with crusty bread

Large green salad

Honeyed apples

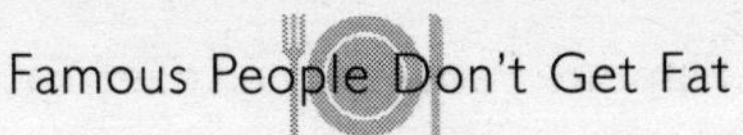

DAY 3

BREAKFAST

Fresh figs

Muesli with skimmed milk

Small bread roll with apricot conserve

LUNCH

Green beans à la Grecque

Guiso Ternera (Spanish veal stew)

DINNER

Roast Lamb Castilian Style

Spanish-style Courgettes

Spanish Fruit Medley

DAY 4

BREAKFAST

Fresh orange juice

Cucumber and ham omelette

Toast

LUNCH

Arroz con Pollo (Spanish chicken and rice)

Large green salad

DINNER

Espinacas con Huevos (spinach with hard-boiled eggs)

Hake with Clams and Peas

Ananas Glacé (pineapple ice dessert)

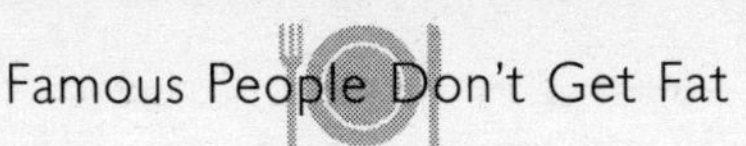

DAY 5

BREAKFAST

Moroccan Orange Salad

LUNCH

Avocado Soup

DINNER

Ensalada Serrano (Spanish appetiser salad)

Albondigas (Spanish meat balls) served with Sopa con Bolitas de Carne (tomato sauce)

Fresh fruit

Salt may cause your body to retain water, giving you that bloated feeling, so follow actress *Jessica Biel's* lead and read the labels on processed foods and look for low-salt options.

Research shows that that people who don't eat breakfast are more likely to be overweight. *Paris Hilton* regularly enjoys a bowl of porridge first thing in the morning as it keeps her feeling full until lunch.

Tortilla

(Makes 6 slices)

2 tablespoons olive oil

125g diced ham

1 large potato peeled and diced

½ large Spanish onion, peeled and chopped

6 eggs, well beaten

salt and freshly ground black pepper

additional olive oil

Heat the olive oil in a large omelette pan. Add the diced ham, diced potato and chopped onion and cook until the onion and potato are soft. Season the eggs with salt and pepper and pour one third of the mixture into the pan, lifting up with a spatula to allow the egg to run underneath the ham and vegetables. Add the remainder of the eggs and continue to cook until the omelette has a golden crust on the bottom.

Now place a large plate on the omelette pan and invert the pan so that the omelette is on the plate crust-side up. Scrape free any crusty bits from pan, add a little more olive oil, return the omelette to the pan moist side down, and continue to cook until it has browned on both sides. Cut into wedges and serve with slices of fresh tomoto.

Gazpacho

(Serves 4)

250ml tomato juice
125ml iced water
6 tablespoons olive oil
2–3 tablespoons lemon juice
1 clove garlic
960g ripe tomatoes, peeled, seeded and chopped
1 cucumber, peeled and chopped
½ large Spanish onion, finely chopped
salt and freshly ground black pepper
cayenne pepper

For the garnish

½ green pepper, diced
4 slices white bread, diced and sautéed in butter and olive oil until crisp and golden
1 avocado, peeled, stoned, diced and brushed with lemon juice to preserve colour
4 tablespoons coarsely chopped parsley

Combine the tomato juice, iced water, olive oil and lemon juice in a large tureen or serving bowl which you have rubbed with garlic. Add the tomatoes (be sure to add all the juice), cucumber and onion, and generous amounts of salt and pepper, and cayenne, to taste. Chill thoroughly.

Serve the soup in individual soup bowls with an ice cube in each bowl and a crusty wholemeal roll on the side. Garnish with a sprinkling of diced green pepper, croutons, diced avocado and chopped parsley.

Cauliflower Salad Niçoise

(Serves 6)

1 cauliflower
6 anchovy fillets, finely chopped
12 black olives, pitted and finely chopped
3 tablespoons finely chopped parsley
1 clove garlic, finely chopped
1 tablespoon finely chopped capers
6 tablespoons olive oil
2 tablespoons wine vinegar
6 medium tomatoes, halved, to garnish
salt and freshly ground black pepper

Trim the outer leaves of the cauliflower and trim the stem. Break into florets and poach in lightly salted water for about 5 minutes. Drain well. Mix the anchovies, olives, parsley, garlic and capers with oil and vinegar in a large mixing bowl and add the cauliflower, seasoning to taste with salt and freshly ground black pepper. To serve, arrange the marinated cauliflower and dressing in a salad dish and garnish with tomato around the sides.

Chuletas

(Serves 4-6)

4–6 sirloin steaks, 2cm thick

6 tablespoons olive oil

4 tablespoons dry white wine

1 tablespoon lemon juice

2 tablespoons coarsely chopped Spanish onion

2 cloves garlic, chopped

¼ teaspoon dried oregano

½ teaspoon crumbled bay leaves

1 tablespoon chopped parsley

salt and freshly ground black pepper

Pierce the steaks all over with a thick barbeque skewer. Combine the remaining ingredients in a bowl and cover the steaks with this mixture, forcing it well down into the holes in the meat. Allow to marinate for at least 2 hours before cooking. Heat the grill until very hot, place steaks on the grill pan and brush with the marinade. Grill for 5 minutes on each side for a rare steak; grill a few minutes longer if you prefer it to be medium rare.

Higos Borrachos

(Serves 4)

8–12 fresh figs, or 1 large can figs, drained
¼ teaspoon ground cinnamon
1 tablespoon grated orange rind
2 tablespoons brandy
4 tablespoons sherry
icing sugar, if desired

Combine the cinnamon, orange rind, brandy and sherry and sprinkle over the figs with a little icing sugar. Allow the figs to marinate in this flavouring for at least 1 hour before serving.

Revelto con Setas

(Serves 4)

8 eggs

4 tablespoons milk

60g butter

200g mushrooms (wild if possible)

lemon juice

salt and freshly ground black pepper

Clean the mushrooms and slice thinly. Melt 20g of the butter in a pan, add the mushrooms, a few drops of lemon juice and a little salt and cook for about 5 minutes or until the liquid has been driven off. Break the eggs into a bowl and whisk. Add the eggs to the mushrooms together with the remaining butter, seasoning with salt and pepper to taste, stirring until the eggs are cooked through. Serve with some crusty bread.

Baked Fish Spanish Style

(Serves 6)

3lbs cod, hake or halibut

For the tomato sauce

1 Spanish onion, chopped

2 tablespoons olive oil

1 tin tomatoes

150ml dry white wine

2 cloves

1 level tablespoon cornflour

1 tablespoon water

12 green olives, pitted and cut into pieces

1 tablespoon chopped parsley

2 level tablespoons capers

salt and freshly ground pepper

Sauté the onion in the oil until soft, then add the tomatoes, wine, cloves and seasoning. Cover the pan and simmer for 20 minutes. Blend the cornflour with the water to a smooth paste and stir into the mixture. Simmer for 5 minutes then add the olives, parsley and capers.

Wash and dry the fish and place in a well-greased baking dish. Pour the tomato sauce over it and bake in a preheated moderate oven for 35 minutes or until the fish flakes easily with a fork. Baste occasionally. Serve hot with a green salad dressed with lemon juice.

Paella

(Serves 6)

12 mussels in their shells
6 tablespoons dry white wine
2 tablespoons finely chopped onion
4 tablespoons finely chopped parsley
1 free range chicken, cut into 8 portions
250g lean pork, diced
125g chorizo sausage, sliced
150ml light olive oil
1 small cooked lobster, cut into pieces
8 large raw whole prawns
1 Spanish onion finely chopped
4 cloves garlic, finely chopped
4 large ripe tomatoes, peeled and chopped
2 tinned pimentos, cut into strips
¼ teaspoon cayenne powder
½ teaspoon powdered saffron
450ml boiling chicken stock
480g uncooked risotto rice
salt and freshly ground black pepper

Steam the mussels in the white wine with 2 tablespoons each of the finely chopped onion and parsley until the shells open. Put the mussels to one side. Strain the liquor and reserve.

Sauté the chicken, pork and sausage in olive oil in a paella pan or large frying pan until golden on all sides. Remove and reserve. Sauté prawns in the same pan and reserve. Add the Spanish onion and 2 chopped cloves of garlic to the pan and sauté until transparent. Add the tomatoes and pimento and simmer the mixture for about 5 minutes stirring constantly. Return the chicken, pork, sausage, half the lobster, the prawns and the mussels to the pan. Add the mussel liquor, season to taste with salt, pepper and cayenne pepper and heat through.

Mix the remaining garlic, parsley and powdered saffron in 1 cup of boiling stock, add to remaining stock and pour over the meat and seafood mixture. Stir well and slowly bring to the boil again. Pour over the rice and cook, uncovered, for 20 minutes without stirring. Stir well with a wooden spoon. Garnish with the remaining lobster, prawns and mussels. Cook for 10 to 15 minutes or until the rice is tender, adding a little more boiling stock if necessary. Serve with green salad and crusty bread.

Honeyed Apples

(Serves 6)

60g dried figs

30g blanched almonds, chopped

3 tablespoons water

120g honey

1 teaspoon melted butter

6 medium-sized apples

Pre-heat the oven to 160°C/gas mark 3. Mix the figs and almonds together. In another small bowl stir together the water, honey and butter. Twist the stems from the apples, then starting at the other end, peel each apple about a third of the way down. Remove the cores part way down. Fill the apples with the fig and almond mixture, arrange them in a shallow baking dish and pour on the water and honey.

Bake in the centre of the oven, basting frequently with the syrup until tender but still unbroken, about 1¼ hours. Refrigerate until required.

Green beans à la Grecque

(Serves 6)

480g green beans

1 medium tin tomato concentrate

600ml water

4–6 tablespoons olive oil

½ Spanish onion, finely chopped

1 clove garlic, finely chopped

salt and freshly ground black pepper

chopped parsley

Top and tail the beans and slice them in half lengthways. Mix the tomato concentrate with the water, olive oil, onion and garlic. Put the beans into a saucepan, pour over the tomato mixture and season to taste. Bring to the boil. Lower the heat and simmer gently, stirring from time to time, for 45 minutes until sauce has reduced and the beans are tender. Garnish with the parsley.

Guiso Ternera

(Serves 6)

960g shoulder of veal

flour

5 tablespoons olive oil

2 Spanish onions, chopped

2 cloves garlic, chopped

8 stalks celery (about 5cm long)

8 thick 5cm strips green pepper

2 bay leaves

2 sprigs thyme

300ml dry white wine

salt and freshly ground black pepper

Cut the veal into 4cm cubes. Season with salt and pepper, dust with flour and sauté in the olive oil in a large heatproof casserole until well browned. Remove the meat. Add the finely chopped onion and garlic to the casserole and sauté, adding more oil if necessary. Stir constantly until soft. Add the celery, green pepper, bay leaves and thyme and simmer for a few minutes longer. Pour in the wine and stir.

Cover the casserole and simmer gently for about 1½ hours or until the meat is tender, adding a little hot water from time to time if the stew seems too dry.

Roast Lamb Castilian Style

(Serves 6)

1.5 kg leg of lamb
2 tablespoons olive oil
1 teaspoon fresh thyme leaves
2 cloves garlic, finely sliced
1 wineglass of dry white wine
300ml water
2 tablespoons wine vinegar
juice of 1 lemon
960g potatoes
2 large onions
5 whole garlic cloves.
salt and freshly ground black pepper

Pre-heat the oven to 230°C/gas mark 8. Rub the lamb with half of the oil, season it with salt and pepper then rub the thyme over the surface of the lamb. Let the lamb sit for an hour to absorb the flavours.

Peel and cut the potatoes into slices about 1cm thick

and place on the bottom of a roasting tin. Slice the onions and mix them with the potatoes. Peel the garlic, leaving them whole and add to the potatoes and onions.

Put the white wine, water, vinegar and lemon juice into a pan and bring to the boil. Make some slits in the lamb and put the slices of garlic into them, then rub the lamb with the rest of the olive oil. Place the lamb on top of the potatoes, onions and garlic and pour about half of the liquid over the meat. Place in the hot oven for 15 minutes. Turn the heat down to 190°C/gas mark 5 and continue to roast. Baste with the remaining liquid from time to time. If the potatoes soak up all the liquid you can make another batch. Allow 15 minutes per 450g if you like your lamb pink, and 25 minutes per 450g if you like it well done – which is how the Spanish would eat it!

Traditionally in Spain, the lamb would be served with the potato that is cooked alongside it, but you might choose to serve with some other vegetables.

Spanish-style Courgettes

(Serves 6)

10 courgettes
flour
freshly grated Parmesan cheese
olive oil
chopped fresh tomatoes
salt and freshly ground black pepper

Boil the whole courgettes in salted water until just tender. Do not let them lose their shape. Cut in thick slices, dust with seasoned flour and then roll in grated Parmesan cheese. Fry in hot oil until golden brown on both sides. Place on kitchen paper to remove excess fat and serve hot with chopped fresh tomatoes.

Cucumber and Ham Omelette

(Serves 3)

3 tablespoons peeled, seeded and diced cucumber

butter

3 tablespoons diced cooked ham

1 teaspoon finely chopped chives

salt and freshly ground black pepper

6 eggs, well beaten

Drop the diced cucumber into boiling salted water and boil for 3 minutes. Drain well and dry with kitchen paper. Melt 2 tablespoons of butter and sauté the diced cucumber and ham for 5 minutes, stirring constantly. Add the chives and season to taste. Combine the mixture with the eggs and make the omelette in the usual way.

Arroz con Pollo

(Serves 6)

2 young free-range chickens
8 tablespoons light olive oil
½ Spanish onion, finely chopped
6 tablespoons well-flavoured tomato sauce
¼ teaspoon powdered saffron
600ml well-flavoured chicken stock
180g rice
2 canned pimentos, sliced
grated rind of ½ lemon
2 tablespoons freshly chopped parsley
salt and freshly ground black pepper

Cut each chicken into serving portions, season and sauté in olive oil until golden on all sides. Stir in the onion and garlic and continue to cook until soft – don't let the onions go brown. Add the tomato sauce, saffron, sliced pimentos and chicken stock. Cover the saucepan and simmer for 15 minutes.

Stir the rice into the chicken and vegetable mixture, season with salt and freshly ground black pepper. Cover the saucepan again and simmer for 30 minutes, or until all the liquids have been absorbed and the chicken is tender. Sprinkle with grated lemon rind and chopped parsley. Serve with green salad.

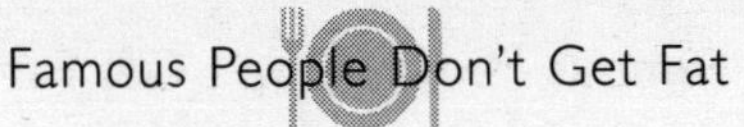

Espinacas con Huevos

(Serves 2)

960g fresh spinach

4 tablespoons olive oil

2 small cloves of very finely chopped garlic

2 eggs, hard-boiled and sliced

2 canned pimentos cut in strips

salt and freshly ground pepper

Wash the spinach in several changes of water and drain. Place in a thick-bottomed saucepan with the olive oil. Season to taste with salt, pepper and garlic. Cook over a fairly high heat, stirring constantly until the spinach is soft and wilted. Transfer spinach to a heated serving dish. Top with slices of hard-boiled egg and strips of pimento.

Ananas Glacé

(Serves 4)

4 slices fresh pineapple

4 medium oranges, peeled and segmented

4 scoops vanilla ice cream

Chocolate curls

Remove the hard central core from a fresh pineapple and cut into 4 equal slices. Arrange on a plate and add the orange segments in a flower shape on the top. Just before serving place a scoop of ice cream in the hollow of the pineapple. Sprinkle with the chocolate curls.

Moroccan Orange Salad

(Serves 6)

6 ripe oranges

6 dates, chopped

6 blanched almonds, slivered

orange flower water (or lemon juice and powdered sugar)

powdered cinnamon

Peel the oranges, removing all pith, and slice crossways. Place in a salad bowl with the dates and almonds and flavour to taste with the orange flower water. Chill. Just before serving sprinkle lightly with powdered cinnamon.

Avocado Soup

(Serves 6)

3 ripe avocado pears

1½ teaspoons curry powder

175ml double cream

900ml good vegetable or chicken stock

3 teaspoons lemon juice

cayenne pepper

salt and freshly ground pepper

finely chopped coriander or parsley

Peel the avocados thinly and halve each one lengthwise; remove stones and dice flesh, retaining a little of the darker green flesh for garnish. Blend the diced avocado in an electric blender together with the curry powder, salt and pepper and double cream.

In a saucepan, combine the stock and lemon juice. Bring gently to the boil, then remove from the heat and add a little to the avocado and cream mixture. Blend all together with the remaining stock and reheat gently. Correct the seasoning, adding a little cayenne pepper and more lemon juice if desired. Serve in individual bowls, garnished with chunks of dark green avocado and a sprinkling of finely chopped herbs.

Ensalada Serrano

(Serves 6)

720g new potatoes, boiled

1 large can tuna

12 black olives

12 green olives

2 hard-boiled eggs, sliced

For the dressing

3 tablespoons wine vinegar

8 tablespoons olive oil

¼ teaspoon each of poppy seeds, sesame seeds and celery seeds

salt and freshly ground black pepper

Mix the dressing ingredients together. Peel and slice the potatoes. Toss lightly in half the dressing and arrange in a shallow salad bowl. Drain the fish and break into chunks. Place on top of the potatoes. Garnish the dish with the olives and hard-boiled eggs. Pour over the remaining dressing and serve immediately.

Albondigas

(Serves 6)

960g lean minced beef

¼ Spanish onion, finely chopped

olive oil

4 tablespoons fresh breadcrumbs

2 level teaspoons salt

¼ teaspoon rubbed thyme

¼ teaspoon cayenne pepper

1 bay leaf, crumbled

grated rind of ½ lemon

2 eggs

Place the beef in a large mixing bowl. Sauté the onion in 4 tablespoons of olive oil until soft and add to the meat, mixing well. Add the breadcrumbs, salt, thyme, cayenne, crumbled bay leaf and grated lemon rind. Mix well. Beat the eggs, add to the meat mixture and thoroughly combine. Allow the flavours to blend for 20 minutes, adding additional salt, pepper, thyme or lemon rind to taste. Form into little balls the size of walnuts. Place the albondigas in the refrigerator to firm. When ready to serve sauté gently in olive oil until cooked through.

Sopa con Bolitas de Carne

(Serves 6)

900ml well-flavoured beef stock

½ tin tomatoes

1 bay leaf

1 Spanish onion, finely chopped

1 fat clove garlic, finely chopped

2 tablespoons olive oil

Combine the stock, tomatoes and bay leaf in a large saucepan. Bring to the boil, skim and simmer gently for 10 minutes. In a separate pan, sauté the onion and garlic in olive oil until soft, then add to the stock and continue to cook for 10 minutes.

To serve, either add the cooked albondigas to the sauce and heat through gently in a covered pan, or serve the sauce separately.

Halle Berry

WAS THERE a single woman who saw Halle Berry emerge from the sea in the hit Bond movie *Die Another Day* and didn't dream of having the flat tummy and voluptuous curves that ensnared 007 in a matter of seconds?

But Halle's slimming secrets couldn't be much simpler. Why not follow them to get the body *you've* been dreaming about? First rule is to cut out sugar. Halle was diagnosed as a diabetic at the age of 19 and, although she has managed to control the condition, she now hardly eats any refined sugar, preferring to stick to the natural – and much more healthy – sugars that are found in fruit and vegetables.

Rule number two: cut out fried foods. It's as simple as that.

Halle's third slimming tip is to eat at home, where you can control what you're eating, rather than eating out in restaurants. Of course, there are times when you just can't avoid restaurants – when this is the case, see page 304 for tips on cutting down the calories when eating out.

And finally, Halle never eats after 7 pm – a fantastic slimming tip, as there's nothing worse for the committed dieter than going to bed on a full stomach. Eat earlier and you'll have a chance to burn off those calories before getting your beauty sleep.

Lynda Carter

AS YOU would expect of Wonder Woman herself, Lynda Carter's slimming secrets are a bit more adventurous than most. Not for her the daily grind of calorie watching and portion control – although we suspect that even superheroes would put on weight if they ate nothing but burgers and fries! Lynda likes to stay slim by keeping her body in good shape. But if you think that has to mean gruelling sessions in the gym, think again…

Lynda's approach is only to do exercise that she enjoys – skiing, for example, or skating. It's a great way to keep you interested in exercising, which, let's face it, can become a bit dull after a while. Why not try a scenic cycle ride or a sociable game of tennis? Even if you are a gym fanatic, you can liven up those sessions by concentrating on getting yourself fit for your favourite sports. Here are a few ideas about how to get fit, lose weight and have fun, all at the same time – just like Lynda:

SWIMMING

Swimming is almost the perfect exercise. Unlike most other popular sports, it uses nearly all the major muscle groups, increases your flexibility and gets your aerobic fitness up to scratch. It also avoids stress to your knee and ankle joints, which can be a problem with other sports if you are a little overweight.

The key to enjoying your swimming sessions is to build up your fitness levels gradually. Work out how many times a week you can go swimming, and gradually build up the number of lengths you do, or the amount of time you swim, each time you go. Write yourself an exercise plan – you know what is realistic for your personal level of fitness, but try to push yourself a little bit further every time you go. Your exercise plan might look like this:

WEEK 1	
Tuesday	10 lengths
Thursday	12 lengths
Saturday	14 lengths
WEEK 2	
Tuesday	16 lengths
Thursday	18 lengths
Saturday	20 lengths

And so on. If you can reach a stage where you are swimming for 45 minutes three times every week, you will be amazed at how you start to keep your weight down – and you will feel absolutely fantastic.

SKIING

If you are lucky enough to be able to indulge in a skiing holiday now and then, you can get prepared to have fun and lose weight all at the same time. You need to increase your flexibility, strength and general aerobic fitness – this will have the double advantage of making you look like a whiz on the slopes and keeping your figure in trim. In addition, the fitter you are, the less likely you are to sustain any kind of injury.

Try to start building up your fitness levels at least six weeks before you go on your skiing holiday. If your local gym does step and aerobics classes, go two or three times a week. Build flexibility by doing gentle stretches every day; and if you have access to the proper machines, build up your muscle strength by doing leg presses, bench presses, squats and abdominal crunches three times a week. If you've never done this before, make sure you do so under supervision – most good gyms will have someone who will show you the ropes and devise a fitness regime for you.

At the end of six weeks you'll be fit enough to enjoy your holiday to the full, and you'll be amazed at how much slimmer you've become!

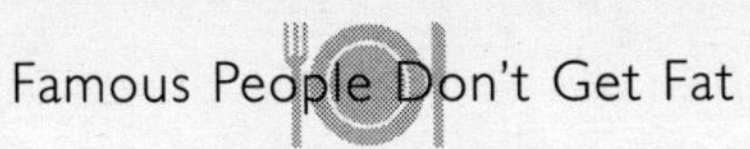

CYCLING

Cycling can be so much fun that it hardly even feels like exercising. Again, because it has little impact on the knees and ankles, it is particularly good if you are slightly overweight.

A half-hour recreational cycle ride three times a week will start to achieve weight loss very quickly indeed. But even better, if it's possible for you, why not cycle to work? Riding there and back five times a week may well be the best exercise, and the most effective weight-loss programme, you've ever done.

One word of caution – wherever you plan to cycle, and especially in the city, get yourself a good-quality cycling helmet.

Courtney Cox knows that white bread, pasta and rice can cause bloating and weight gain. She eats wholemeal foods which help balance blood sugars and reduce cravings – and help maintain her svelte figure!

Cindy Crawford

LET'S FACE it. If a diet's good enough for Cindy, then it's good enough for the rest of us. Supermodels, of course, make a career out of looking great, so it's hardly surprising that they have a fund of tips and secrets to help them keep those fantastic figures. Did you know, for example, that supermodels make a point of sipping ice-cold water throughout the day because the body uses up calories to warm it up?

Cindy has said that she avoids dairy products as she finds these can pile on the weight, and of course it is true that cheese, milk and cream are a dieter's worst enemy. There are plenty of ways that you can cut down on your intake of dairy products. Here are a few of them:

- Use a low-calorie coffee whitener instead of milk or cream.
- If you don't like black tea, try herbal teas, which have their own health benefits (see page 2).
- Low-fat yogurt can be a great substitute for cream in all sorts of sauces.
- If you really love your milk, always buy the skimmed version – it contains all the nutrients and much less of the fat.

Remember, if you cut out dairy products, you must make sure you are getting enough calcium, perhaps in the form of supplements, to keep your bone structure healthy and avoid osteoporosis in later life.

Cindy is also an advocate of the popular high-protein, low-carbohydrate diets – see the appendix.

Jamie Lee Curtis

SULTRY JAMIE Lee has sizzled on our screens in any number of big Hollywood movies. But that incredible figure doesn't come naturally. Even Jamie is subject to the ups and downs of her weight, and to counteract this she has been known to completely ban fat from her diet and eat only fresh vegetables.

And if that sounds like it might not be the most exciting way to eat, it needn't be dull. Have a go at some of these delicious fat-free and low-fat vegetable dishes, and maybe you can have a figure like Jamie's.

Satisfying Spinach Salad

(Serves 1)

3 handfuls baby spinach, washed and with stalks removed

a handful of watercress, washed and with stalks removed

¼ cucumber, peeled

1 tablespoon lime juice

½ teaspoon French mustard

6 radishes, sliced

Liquidise the cucumber, lime juice and mustard, thinning with a little water if necessary. Pour this over the spinach and cress, garnish with the radishes and serve.

Colourful Vegetable Dish in their Own Sweet Sauce

(Serves 4)

5 leeks, washed and sliced into thin rounds

2 large yellow peppers, halved, deseeded and sliced

1 large red pepper, halved, deseeded and sliced

40g butter

1 tablespoon virgin olive oil

1½ tablespoons fresh mixed herbs, chopped

salt and white pepper

Melt the butter in a pan with 3 tablespoons of water, then add the leeks and a little salt. Cover the pan and cook over a medium heat for about 8 minutes until tender. Uncover the pan, add the oil and increase the heat. Sauté the peppers for 2 minutes. Add a little more water, reduce the heat and cook for a further 2 minutes until the peppers are soft and there is a sweet sauce in the pan. Add the herbs, season with salt and pepper, and serve.

Casserole of Braised Vegetables

(Serves 4)

25g dried mushrooms
1 medium onion, peeled and thinly sliced
2–3 garlic cloves, peeled and thinly sliced
15 small shallots, peeled
12 baby carrots, peeled
3 parsnips, peeled, quartered, cored and cut into 25mm lengths
175g fresh chestnut mushrooms, wiped and halved
4 baby cauliflowers, broken into florets
8 Brussels sprouts, trimmed and halved
1 celeriac root, cut into 50mm x 15mm pieces
225g green beans, topped and tailed
75g frozen peas, thawed
40g butter
1½ tablespoons virgin olive oil
1 bay leaf
2 tablespoons fresh herbs, chopped
1 small glass dry white wine
salt and freshly ground black pepper

Soak the dried mushrooms according to the packet instructions. Reserve the soaking water.

Melt 25g of the butter in a large casserole dish with 1 tablespoon of the olive oil. Add the sliced onion, cover and cook for 2–3 minutes. Add the shallots and carrots and cook for 5 minutes. Add the garlic, the bay leaf, a pinch of salt and a pinch of the fresh herbs, and cook for 3 minutes. Add the celeriac, parsnips and another pinch of salt and herbs and cook for 6–10 minutes until tender but crisp.

Heat the remaining butter and olive oil in a pan, then add the fresh mushrooms. Sauté these over a medium to high heat until the juices run, then add the dried mushrooms and reserved juices and the wine. Cover the pan and simmer for 3 minutes before adding to the casserole.

Add the green beans and peas to the casserole and cook for 3 minutes. Remove the bay leaf, season with salt and pepper, and add the remaining herbs. Serve immediately.

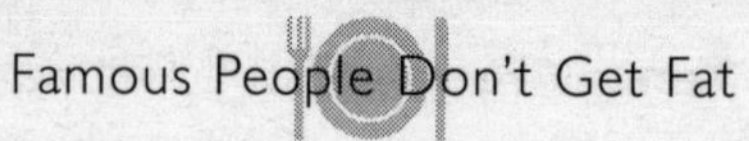

Far Eastern Vegetables Flavoured with Orange

(Serves 4)

115g daikon (or mooli), cut into strips

115g carrots, cut into strips

2 sticks celery, cut into strips

½ green pepper, cut into strips

4 spring onions, cut into strips

25mm fresh root ginger

2 garlic cloves

225g packet thread noodles

2 tablespoons vegetable oil

115g bean sprouts

salt and freshly ground black pepper

SAUCE

4 tablespoons orange juice

2 tablespoons shoyu

2 tablespoons clear honey

1 tablespoon cider vinegar

1 tablespoon dry sherry

1 tablespoon cornflour

1 teaspoon tomato purée

Keep each of the cut vegetables and the bean sprouts in separate piles. Finely chop the ginger and peel and crush the garlic. Mix the sauce ingredients in a bowl and put aside. Add the noodles to a pan of salted, boiling water and cook according to the instructions on the packet.

Heat a wok, add the oil and heat until hot, then add the spring onions and ginger and stir-fry for 2 minutes until soft, being careful not to burn them. Add the daikon, carrots and garlic and stir-fry for a further 2 minutes leaving them still crisp.

Add the celery and green pepper and stir-fry for 2 minutes. Add the bean sprouts and continue cooking for a further 2 minutes. Stir the sauce and pour it over the vegetables. Add the drained noodles and toss until evenly combined and heated through. Season and serve immediately.

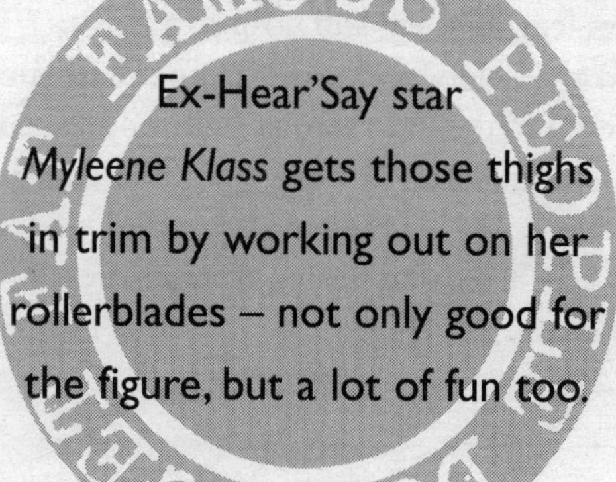

Ex-Hear'Say star *Myleene Klass* gets those thighs in trim by working out on her rollerblades – not only good for the figure, but a lot of fun too.

Baby Spice *Emma Bunton* keeps her A-list figure in trim by regular detox sessions, massages and detox baths to shift those harmful toxins.

Spring Ratatouille

(Serves 4)

2 tablespoons virgin olive oil
4 tomatoes, skinned and sliced
1 large aubergine, sliced
3 medium courgettes, sliced
1 medium red pepper, sliced
2 red onions, skinned and sliced
½ cucumber, sliced
2 large garlic cloves, crushed
parsley, chopped
salt and freshly ground black pepper

Heat the oven to 175°C/gas mark 4. Heat the oil in a flameproof casserole and add the prepared vegetables, garlic, salt and pepper. Stir well, cover tightly and cook in the oven for 1–1¼ hours. Serve garnished with the parsley. This dish is also delicious served cold.

Vegetable Strudel

(Serves 4 – could be a main course)

8 sheets filo pastry
2 sticks celery, thinly sliced
115g courgettes, thinly sliced
4 spring onions, thinly sliced
2 carrots, peeled and thinly sliced
115g button mushrooms, thinly sliced
1 orange pepper, halved, deseeded and sliced
50g mangetout, topped and tailed and sliced
50g frozen sweetcorn, thawed and drained
115g bean sprouts, soaked in cold water for 5 minutes and then rinsed
3 tablespoons vegetable oil
50g cashew nuts
1 teaspoon ground ginger
2 teaspoons arrowroot
1 tablespoon light soy sauce
1 tablespoon tomato purée
3 tablespoons cider vinegar
2 tablespoons brown sugar
1 tablespoon sesame seeds

Heat 2 tablespoons of the oil in a wok over a high heat. Add the cashew nuts and cook them briefly, stirring continuously until golden. Leaving the oil in the wok, remove the nuts and put them aside.

Stir-fry the celery and carrots for 2 minutes over a high heat. Add the remaining vegetables one batch at a time, stirring well between each addition, and stir-fry for a total of 4 minutes.

Combine the ground ginger, arrowroot, soy sauce, tomato purée, cider vinegar and sugar, and mix well. Add the mixture to the wok and cook for 2 minutes, stirring well, until thickened. Transfer it to a bowl and leave to cool.

Lay 2 sheets of the filo pastry, slightly overlapping, on a clean work surface. Lay the next 2 sheets on top, with the pastry seam lying in the opposite direction. Repeat the process with the next 2 sheets in the original direction and the last 2 in the opposite direction. You should have a square of pastry with each side measuring about 460mm.

Carefully spread all the vegetable mixture over the pastry, leaving a 25mm space around the edges. Fold in two sides of the pastry, then carefully roll up the strudel. Transfer to a lightly oiled baking tray. Brush the strudel with the remaining oil and sprinkle with the sesame seeds. Bake in the oven for about 30 minutes until golden brown. Allow to cool for 5 minutes, then cut into thick slices and serve.

Broad Beans with Dill Sauce

(Serves 4)

240g frozen broad beans

285ml vegetable stock

½ tablespoon dill, chopped

15g unsalted butter

1 teaspoon arrowroot

salt and freshly ground black pepper

Cook the broad beans gently in the stock and strain, reserving the stock. Return the stock to the pan with half the dill and the butter. Mix the arrowroot with 2 tablespoons of water and add to the pan, stirring occasionally until it is reduced to a glaze.

Return the vegetables to the pan with the remainder of the dill and season with salt and pepper.

Cameron Diaz swaps coffee for herbal teas – caffeine can slow your metabolism, stimulate your appetite and disrupt sleeping patterns, which can all lead to rapid weight gain.

Sophie Dahl

FOOD-COMBINING diets have been around for a very long time, and stunning Sophie Dahl is one of their more famous exponents. Sophie keeps herself trim by simply avoiding the combination of proteins and carbohydrates in any one meal. You can aim for a body like Sophie's by following these simple rules:

- Don't mix protein and carbohydrate in the same meal.
- Eat at least one protein and one carbohydrate meal per day.

- Eat plenty of vegetables and salad with each meal.

It's as simple as that! Not only can food combining help you lose weight, but it's also often used by people with allergies and skin complaints and can be remarkably effective. And Sophie Dahl is not the only celebrity to follow this eating plan – Koo Stark and Liz Hurley are also reportedly followers of food-combining diets. So why not try these tempting recipes to get a celebrity glow like Sophie (or Koo or Liz!)?

MENU 1

BREAKFAST

Bacon and egg

LUNCH

Bowl watercress soup

Pasta with tomato sauce

1 large slice melon

DINNER

Large salad of lettuce, cucumber, peppers, celery, orange and apple, topped with bean sprouts and freshly chopped herbs

Baked bananas

MENU 2

BREAKFAST

2 slices wholemeal toast with grilled tomatoes

LUNCH

Grilled chicken breast stuffed with cheese

DINNER

Risotto with roasted peppers, courgettes, aubergines and tomatoes

Fresh fruit salad

MENU 3

BREAKFAST

Poached haddock topped with a poached egg

LUNCH

Ratatouille (see page 103) and 2 slices wholemeal bread

2 peaches

DINNER

Medium grilled steak

MENU 4

BREAKFAST

Large bowl porridge with prunes

LUNCH

Grilled salmon

DINNER

Vegetable soup (made with fresh vegetables and vegetable stock Penne with green pesto made with garlic, oil, basil and parsley (but no pine nuts)

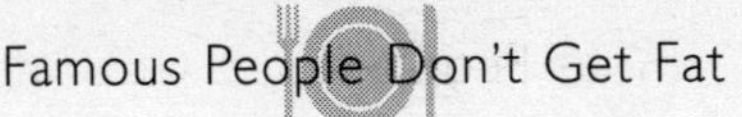

MENU 5

BREAKFAST

2 slices wholemeal toast topped with grilled mushrooms

Banana

LUNCH

Baked halibut, topped with grated cheese and grilled

DINNER

Avocado with vinaigrette

Rice flavoured with saffron mixed with peas, sweetcorn and chopped mixed fresh herbs

Baked apple

When pregnant with her first child, *Charlotte Church's* nesting instinct went into overdrive as she became a cleaning freak – which helped to keep her active right up until the day she gave birth!

Anne Diamond

CELEBRITY TV presenter Anne Diamond's weight soared when she underwent a personal crisis, but she managed to get her life back on track and lose an amazing 25kg with a diet plan that limited her to eating only meals that were no larger than her fist! It might sound a little eccentric, but it is a good way of making sure that you keep an eye on your portion control – one of the most important aspects of any diet.

Here are a few tasty low-fat meals that come under the 'no bigger than your fist' rule:

SEVEN BREAKFASTS

½ grapefruit, 1 slice toast, 1 poached egg

25g porridge with 1 sliced peach

1 slice (25g) toast with 2 grilled tomatoes

1 slice (25g) toast with ½ can sardines in spring water

Compote of 6 prunes, 3 apricots and ½ apple on 25g muesli

1 small banana on 1 slice (25g) toast

1 slice (25g) brown bread with low-fat spread topped with 25g smoked salmon sprinkled with freshly ground black pepper and lemon juice

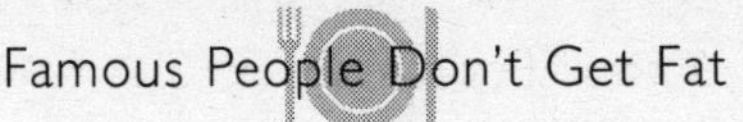

SEVEN MAIN MEALS

50g baked skinless chicken breast with ½ pepper, ½ courgette and ½ onion roasted in 1 teaspoon of olive oil

1 fillet of trout, 1 small (50g) baked potato and 1 grilled tomato

2 cannelloni tubes stuffed with spinach and curd cheese flavoured with nutmeg and seasoning. Serve with a tomato sauce flavoured with oregano and sprinkled with 15g Parmesan cheese

1-egg omelette cooked with 15g grated cheese and served with 1 tomato dressed with French dressing and garnished with chopped chives

50g fillet steak grilled with garlic and served with 1 tablespoon spinach and 2 small new potatoes

1 tablespoon savoury minced beef, 1 tablespoon mashed potatoes, 1 tablespoon cabbage

25g roast lamb, 2 small new potatoes, 1 tablespoon peas served with a little gravy and mint sauce

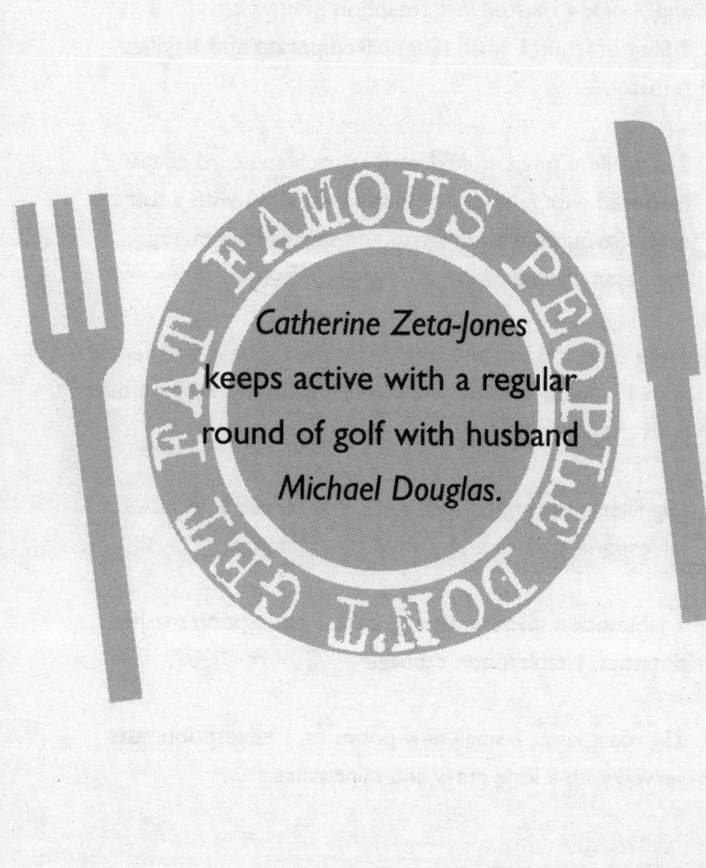
FAMOUS PEOPLE DON'T GET FAT
Catherine Zeta-Jones keeps active with a regular round of golf with husband *Michael Douglas.*

Posh Spice *Victoria Beckham* has her own trampoline which she uses to keep her slim figure even slimmer. Ten minutes on the trampoline is the equivalent of 30 minutes' jogging!

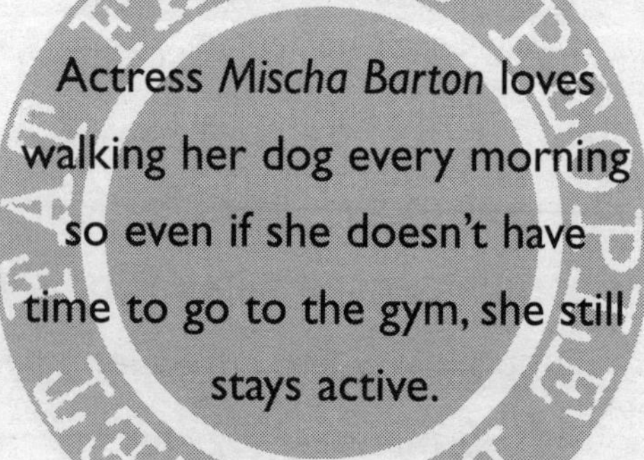

Actress *Mischa Barton* loves walking her dog every morning so even if she doesn't have time to go to the gym, she still stays active.

Cameron Diaz

THERE REALLY is something about Cameron Diaz, and it's not just her brilliant acting skills. Her svelte figure is something that, fortunately for her, she does not have to work on too hard. Cameron has a naturally high metabolism, which means that she burns up any excess calories very easily.

If you are lucky enough to have such a metabolism, then perhaps you find, like Cameron, that it can make you feel not quite your best first thing in the morning. Cameron's solution? To eat a hearty portion of chicken first thing in the morning. It might sound a little strange, but actually it's not such a bad idea. Chicken, cooked in the right way, is low in fat and high in protein; and eating well first thing in the morning is a good slimming technique because it can help you avoid those mid-morning snack attacks.

Here are a couple of good, low-fat chicken recipes to help you on your way – both of which you can, if you want, prepare the night before and then cook in the morning.

Chicken in a Parcel

225g lean chicken breast
2 small tomatoes, sliced
a squeeze of lemon juice
a little fresh tarragon, chopped

Pre-heat the oven to 190°C/gas mark 5. Cut a square of cooking foil large enough to wrap loosely around the chicken breast and place the sliced tomatoes in the middle of the foil. Place the chicken on top, season with lemon juice, tarragon and some salt and pepper, and wrap the foil around it. Scrunch up the foil at the top so that no steam will escape, place on a baking tray and bake for about 20 minutes until the chicken is cooked.

Chicken and Vegetable Kebabs

225g lean breast of chicken, cut into bite-sized pieces

1 small courgette

6 cherry tomatoes

3 shallots, halved

½ red pepper, cut into 6 pieces

½ green pepper, cut into 6 pieces

Thread the ingredients on to two kebab skewers, alternating the ingredients. Spray with a little oil and grill until the chicken is cooked through.

Vanessa Feltz

VANESSA FELTZ'S weight has long been a subject of media interest – and the odd unkind comment. But, amazingly, Vanessa went from a size 26 to a size 12 when she got her figure back on track. Her secrets? Well, there are two. The first was to have an affair with her fitness instructor – unfortunately, not all of us are so lucky!

But Vanessa's great tip for us non-celebrity dieters is a simple but effective one. Eat slowly! Always remember that it takes at least 15 minutes to register that your stomach is full. If you're wolfing your food down, you'll find that you eat more than you actually need – a sure way of putting weight on rather than watching it drop off.

Sarah Michelle Geller

SLINKY, SEXY vampire slayer Buffy certainly needs to keep in trim if she's to keep those evil demons at bay. Actress Sarah Michelle Gellar manages it by cutting out all processed food, all fried food and caffeine.

Sarah's secret ingredient, though, is sushi. Incredibly, fresh raw fish, a little rice, raw vegetables and seaweed can be the dieter's best friend – and Sarah Michelle Gellar has the body to prove it.

She also keeps in trim by practising the martial art of Tae Kwon Do – a great way of keeping in trim and relaxing at the same time – and with regular trampoline and gymnastics sessions.

And when she's not beating up the evil inhabitants of Sunnydale, she keeps that tummy in shape by intensive belly dancing sessions. Did you know that an hour's belly dancing can burn off as many calories as half an hour's intensive aerobics. Not a bad reason for slimming the Buffy way.

Melanie Griffith

WHEN YOU'RE as busy as Melanie Griffith, with a successful career and a family to look after, you don't have time for intricate exercise routines or complicated, time-consuming diet plans. Which isn't to say that Melanie doesn't exercise or watch what she eats – of course she does. She just manages it by keeping it simple.

Melanie's exercise regime revolves around activities that don't require fancy equipment or expensive trainers – running, swimming, walking and running. And her secret dieting weapon? The smoothie! Smoothies are great for anyone trying to keep in trim.

They are low in fat, they give you a real energy boost, and as they are just made from fruit they are very good for you. And, of course, they're really, really delicious. The great thing about smoothies is that you can experiment to your heart's content, and rest assured that the results are going to be delicious. Here are a few ideas to get you started, but feel free to chop and change the ingredients – or invent your own – depending on what you like best.

Strawberry and Banana Smoothie

1 banana
a handful of strawberries, green stalks removed
a couple of ice cubes
a dash of apple juice

Place the banana, strawberries and ice cubes in a blender, and blitz until smooth. Add a little apple juice if you need to thin it out a bit, and then serve.

Fruits of the Forest Smoothie

I banana
a few raspberries, blackcurrants and blackberries
a couple of ice cubes

Blitz everything together in a liquidiser. When smooth, pass through a sieve to get rid of the seeds, and then serve.

Mango and Lime Smoothie

I banana
I mango, peeled and seed removed
juice of half a lime

Blitz everything together in a blender. Taste, and if you feel it needs a bit more lime juice, feel free to add a little. Serve.

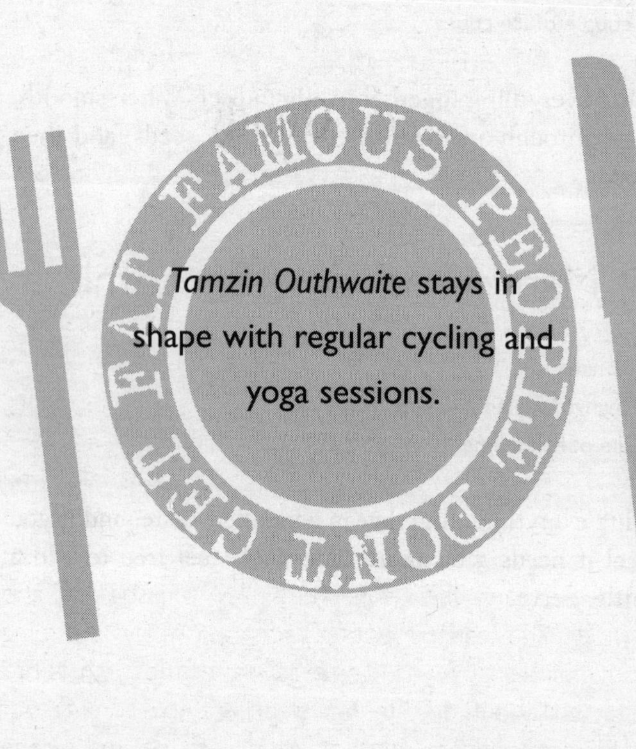

Tamzin Outhwaite stays in shape with regular cycling and yoga sessions.

Jade Goody

BIG BROTHER star Jade Goody certainly earned a reputation for having a big mouth, but the nation loved her for it; she also found it difficult to maintain her size 10 waistline and came out of the series 14 pounds heavier than when she went in. After she left the house, she earned herself admiration for slimming down and shaping up – especially after the birth of her first child. But despite her penchant for coming out with pronouncements that are slightly on the wrong side of outrageous, her slimming secrets are actually rather down-to-earth.

Jade paid a visit to a personal trainer, who instilled in

her the importance of regular exercise if she was to maintain an ideal weight. Jade took the advice on board, and used it to transform herself. Now she is an advocate of the personal-fitness regime she embarked upon, and has even released her own fitness video – a real testament to the fact that if you *want* to lose weight effectively, you *can* do it.

The following fitness regime is based on Jade's. In addition to what is suggested below, you should try and perform three half-hour sessions of cardiovascular exercises every week. These might include jogging, swimming or cycling – try alternating to keep your interest up. As for the following toning exercises, you don't need to invest in expensive gym memberships or equipment – these are all exercises that you can do at home and in your own time. So limber up, and enjoy!

THE WARM-UP

If you have access to an exercise bike, you could spend five or ten minutes using it to warm up, starting at an easy pace and gradually increasing the difficulty over the time of the warm-up. If you don't have a bike, just step up and down the bottom two steps of a staircase for five or ten minutes. But the most important thing to do during your warm-up periods are stretches. In particular, pay attention to doing the following:

HAMSTRING STRETCH

Stretch one leg out in front of you so that your heel is on the floor and your toes are pointing upwards. Keeping your back straight, lean forward and rest your hands on the other knee. Keep it there for a count of twenty, then switch legs.

CALF STRETCH

Face a wall with one leg close to it, knee bent. Place your arm out in front of you and your palm against the wall. Stretch your other leg as far behind you as it will go without lifting your heel or toes from the floor. Keep it there for a count of twenty (slowly!), then switch legs.

FRONT THIGH STRETCH

Stand sideways against a wall and stretch out your arm so that your hand is pressed against the wall. Use your other hand to bring your outside heel up to your bottom. Keep it there for a count of twenty, then switch legs.

THE EXERCISES – CHEST PRESSES

To perform the chest presses, you will need some small weights. If you have a set of dumbbells, great; if not, don't worry – a couple of tins of tomatoes or small bottles of mineral water will do the trick. Lie on your back and extend your arms upwards, holding the weights. The palms of your hands should be facing your feet. Now, slowly lower the weights down to the side until they are just above your shoulders, then slowly arc them back up until they are where they started. Repeat twenty times.

SHOULDER RAISES

Hold a weight in each hand and stand with your feet a foot or so apart. Now slowly raise your arms to the side so that they are at right angles to your body. Keep them there for a second, then slowly lower them. Repeat twenty times.

BICEP CURL

Stand with your feet a foot or so apart. Hold a weight in each hand with your hands by your side. Slowly raise your forearms at the elbow joint until your hands are almost touching your shoulders. Keep you back straight at all times. Slowly move your arms back to their original position. Repeat twenty times.

SQUATS

Stand with your arms at your sides and your feet a foot or so apart. Slowly bend your knees as if you were about to sit down. Keep going until your thighs are just about parallel with the ground. Slowly revert to the standing position. You should concentrate all the time on putting your weight on your heels and not on your toes, and remember that the slower you do this exercise, the better it will be. Repeat fifteen or twenty times.

OUTER THIGH EXERCISES

Lie on your side, using your elbow to support yourself. Place the palm of your other hand on the floor in front of your chest. Bend the knee that is against the floor, then slowly raise your straight leg so that you can feel your outer thigh stretching – about two feet (don't raise it any higher than this). Keep your leg there for a few seconds, then slowly lower it. Repeat fifteen to twenty times, then change sides.

INNER THIGH EXERCISES

Lie on your side, using your elbow to support yourself. Place the palm of your other hand on the floor in front of your chest. Bend the upper leg at the knee and move it up towards your chest; rest your foot on the ground. Point the toes of your straight leg towards your knee, then raise the leg as high as you can without moving your hip off the floor. Keep it there for a few seconds, then slowly lower it. Repeat fifteen to twenty times, then change sides.

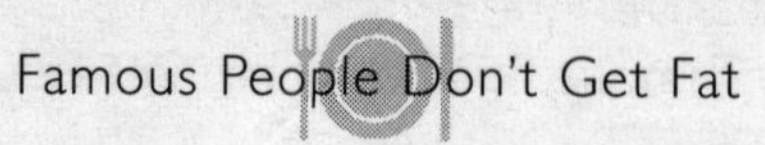

ABDOMINAL CRUNCHES

Lie on your back, then bend your legs so that your feet are flat on the floor. Rest the back of your head on your hands, then curl your body upwards using your stomach muscles – *not* your neck. A good way to make sure you are not using your neck to curl is to find a point on the ceiling and keep your eyes fixed on it. Keep your tummy muscles tensed for a few seconds, then slowly lower yourself back to the ground. Repeat twenty times.

Once you have completed your exercises, you should do a cool-down session. Repeat the warm-up stretches, then do a little light cycling or stepping. And that's all there is too it! Keep plugging away at these exercises and you can experience the amazing weight loss that Jade achieved after she left the *Big Brother* house and became a darling of the celebrity world ...

Geri Halliwell

GERI'S DRAMATIC weight loss caused a sensation all over the world, and everyone wants to know how she managed such a turnaround in her figure. Her well-known adherence to the principles of yoga have certainly helped keep her body in trim. She followed an ancient Indian philosophy called Ayurveda yoga – along with other celebrities, like Sting, Demi Moore and Nicole Kidman. Ayurveda yoga identifies three elements that make up each of us – Vata (air), Pitta (fire) and Kapha (earth). Everyone is a mixture of these three ***doshas***, and unless they are in perfect balance, we can't be in the peak of health and fitness.

Ayurveda yoga practitioners can determine how to keep your *doshas* balanced through a mixture of diet and exercise. (For more information on Ayurveda medicine, see page 335.)

Geri has also tried a number of diets, but the one that works best for her is a customised eating plan that cuts out carbohydrates as far as possible, especially wheat and sugar. And although she has been accused of losing too much weight too fast, this can be a healthy and effective dieting plan if followed sensibly. Here are some recipes that you can follow in order to lose weight by following a similar plan. One word of advice, though. It has been reported that Geri takes vitamin-supplement injections, probably because her exercise regime is so heavy. Healthcare professionals advise that these can cause kidney damage, and so are to be avoided. With this in mind, I have tried to ensure that the following meal plans are well balanced, which means that some of the breakfast options might sound a bit odd! But nothing ventured, nothing gained – and you can always adapt the diet in order to suit your own lifestyle. Just remember: low carb, no wheat, no sugar. (The recipes you need follow the meal plans.)

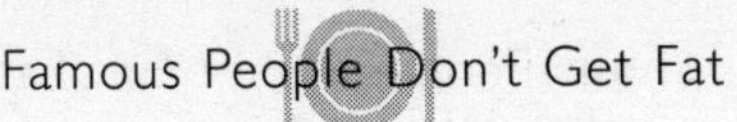

DAY 1

BREAKFAST

180g fresh fruit salad (unsweetened)

LUNCH

Watercress Soup

Smoked Trout Rolls

Strawberry Milkshake

DINNER

Braised Beef

180g broccoli

Medley of Berries

(total calories 838)

DAY 2

BREAKFAST

Artichoke Hearts with Cottage Cheese

LUNCH

Ratatouille

Green salad sprinkled with lemon juice and black pepper

2 satsumas

DINNER

Spicy Chicken with Couscous

Salad of Fruits and Ginger

(total calories 850)

DAY 3

BREAKFAST

Normandy Sausages

LUNCH

Fruit and Vegetable Curry

120g mashed banana and 150ml fat-free yogurt

DINNER

Salmon in a Parcel

Vegetable Rainbow

Florida Cocktail – 115g orange, 115g grapefruit

(total calories 1320)

DAY 4

BREAKFAST

Oriental Combination Salad

LUNCH

Smoked Chicken Salad

90g black grapes

DINNER

Navarin of Lamb

Rhubarb poached in white wine and sweetener

(total calories 1020)

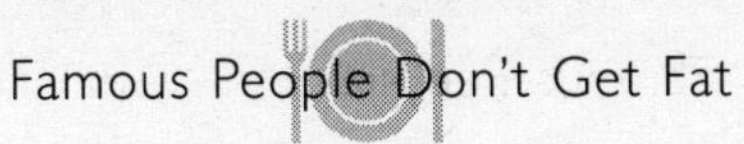

DAY 5

BREAKFAST

Prawn Stir-fry

LUNCH

Exotic Chicken with Spicy Fruits

180g strawberries

DINNER

Roast Loin of Pork with Prunes

180g Brussels sprouts

60g new potatoes

180g raspberries

(total calories 905)

DAY 6

BREAKFAST

120g peeled bananas with 150ml fat-free yogurt

LUNCH

Pea and Ham Risotto

DINNER

Beef Bourguignon

Large green salad

180g pears poached in 150ml red wine and sweetener

(total calories 1105)

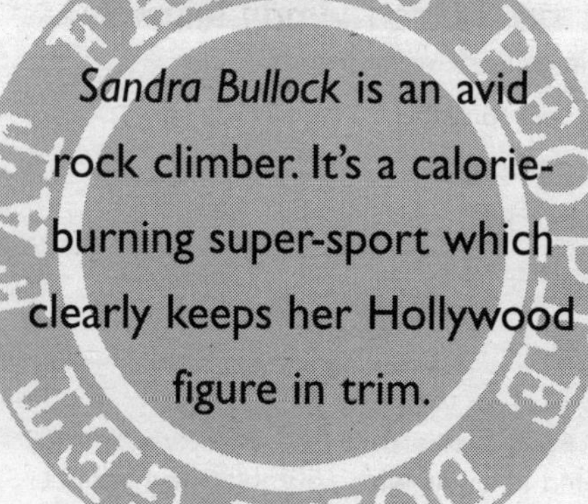

Sandra Bullock is an avid rock climber. It's a calorie-burning super-sport which clearly keeps her Hollywood figure in trim.

Nicole Kidman learned to can-can for the Hollywood blockbuster *Moulin Rouge*. It's one of the most vigorous dances you can do, so if you fancy a Nicole-type figure, why not get those legs moving!

DAY 7

BREAKFAST

2 hard-boiled eggs

60g lean ham

120g fresh pineapple

LUNCH

Parsnip and Apple Soup

Warm Scallop Salad

DINNER

Spicy Kebabs with Cucumber Dip

Green salad with 50g cottage cheese with chives

180g strawberries

(total calories 850)

THE RECIPES

Watercress Soup

(Serves 4)

2 large bunches of watercress
1 medium onion, chopped
450g potatoes, diced
570ml vegetable stock
285ml skimmed milk
¼ teaspoon freshly ground nutmeg
juice of ½ small lemon
1 tablespoon natural yogurt
salt and freshly ground black pepper

Place the onion and potatoes in a large saucepan with the stock, milk and spice. Bring to the boil, then reduce the heat, cover and simmer until the potatoes are tender.

Prepare the watercress and add it with the lemon juice to the saucepan. Remove immediately from the heat and allow it to cool.

Purée the mixture in a liquidiser until smooth. Return to the pan, reheat gently and season with salt and pepper. Swirl a little yogurt into each bowl as you serve.

Smoked Trout Rolls

(Serves 4)

115g smoked trout (you will need 4 good-sized slices)
½ teaspoon powdered gelatine
115g very low-fat cottage cheese
zest of ½ lemon, grated
1 tablespoon lemon juice
1 heaped tablespoon low-fat mayonnaise
2 tablespoons chives, freshly chopped
1 tablespoon dill or fennel, freshly chopped
freshly ground black pepper
dill sprigs and lemon wedges for garnish

In a small bowl, sprinkle the gelatine over 2 tablespoons of water and allow to soak for about 5 minutes until spongy. Drain the cottage cheese and blend to make smooth.

Stand the bowl of gelatine in a saucepan containing hot water to halfway up the bowl. Heat gently until the gelatine is completely dissolved. Do not overheat. Remove the bowl from the water and cool a little.

Stir the gelatine into the cottage cheese and mix thoroughly. Add the finely grated lemon zest, lemon juice, mayonnaise, chopped herbs and pepper and mix thoroughly to make a mousse. Cover and chill in the refrigerator until set. This should take about 1 hour.

Cut each slice of fish in two lengthwise and sprinkle with pepper. Place equal amounts of the mousse at the end of each piece and roll up carefully. Cover and chill.

Garnish the rolls with the dill and lemon and serve on individual plates.

Strawberry Milkshake

(Serves 1)

350g fresh strawberries
a little sweetener if desired
570ml chilled skimmed milk
285ml natural low-fat yogurt
sprig of mint

Put the strawberries in a blender and purée. Add the milk slowly and then the yogurt. Blend at high speed for 1 minute. Serve chilled garnished with mint leaves.

Braised Beef

(Serves 4)

700g boned and rolled very lean brisket of beef
2 large onions, chopped
2 large garlic cloves, crushed
2 tablespoons virgin olive oil
450g large flat mushrooms, roughly chopped
1 tablespoon thyme, freshly chopped
1 tablespoon parsley, freshly chopped
salt and freshly ground black pepper

Heat 1 tablespoon of the oil in a flameproof casserole and quickly brown the meat all over on a high heat. Remove and put aside.

Turn down the heat and add the remainder of the oil. Cook the onions gently for about 5 minutes. Add the garlic, mushrooms and thyme. Mix well, cover the casserole tightly and simmer for about 10 minutes.

Season the mushroom mixture and lay the meat on the top. Cover and cook in a slow oven for about 1 ¾ hours until the meat is tender.

Remove the meat to a heated serving dish and surround with the mushrooms, removing them from the pan with a slotted spoon. Garnish with the parsley. Serve the cooking juices separately.

Medley of Berries

(Serves 4)

115g strawberries

115g raspberries

115g blackberries

115g blueberries

4 tablespoons low-fat yogurt

2 tablespoons Crème de Mur

4 sprigs mint

Divide the yogurt between four plates and sprinkle the Crème de Mur over the top. Arrange the fruits in piles and garnish with the mint.

Artichoke Hearts with Cottage Cheese

(Serves 4)

12 canned small artichoke hearts
juice of 2 small lemons
225g low-fat cottage cheese
2 tablespoons chives, finely chopped
small bag of mixed salad leaves
freshly ground black pepper
parsley sprigs for garnish

DRESSING

1 garlic clove
1 tablespoon white wine vinegar
2 tablespoons parsley, chopped
1 teaspoon Dijon mustard
1 tablespoon virgin olive oil
salt

Drain and rinse the artichoke hearts and mix with the lemon juice. Divide between four plates and fill with the cottage cheese, chives and pepper. Make up the dressing and whisk well. Toss into the salad and serve with the artichokes. Garnish with the parsley.

Ratatouille

(Serves 4)

2 aubergines, peeled
1 red onion, sliced
1 small green pepper, sliced
2 sticks celery, sliced
115g mushrooms, sliced
2 garlic cloves, finely chopped
4 tablespoons extra-virgin olive oil
400g can plum tomatoes
2 tablespoons capers
1 teaspoon dried oregano
50g olives
2 tablespoons wine vinegar
50g pine nuts
salt and freshly ground black pepper

Cut the aubergine into 25mm cubes, put the cubes in a colander with 1 teaspoon of salt and allow to drain for 30 minutes. Rinse the drained aubergine and pat dry.

Heat the oil in a casserole. Sauté the aubergine over a medium heat. Stir constantly until soft and slightly coloured. Remove the aubergines and put aside. Add the onions, garlic, pepper and celery, and cook until quite soft. Chop the tomatoes and add to the pan with the mushrooms and capers. Reduce the heat and simmer for 5 minutes, until the tomato sauce has reduced and thickened. Stir in the aubergines, oregano, olives and wine vinegar.

Simmer for a further 15 minutes, adding a little water if it is too thick. Season with salt and pepper and sprinkle with the pine nuts.

Spicy Chicken with Couscous

(Serves 4–6)

4–6 skinless chicken quarters cut into bite-sized pieces
115g can chickpeas
1 large onion, peeled and thinly sliced
4 medium carrots, cut into thick rounds
4 small turnips, cut into chunks
1 small potato, cut into chunks
2 courgettes, thinly sliced
4 tablespoons virgin olive oil
450g pre-cooked couscous
½ teaspoon ground cinnamon
2 tablespoons seedless raisins
orange-flower water (optional)
salt and freshly ground black pepper
fresh coriander leaves for garnish

SPICE MIXTURE

2 tablespoons tomato purée
2 garlic cloves, crushed
1 teaspoon paprika
1 teaspoon ground cumin
1 teaspoon ground coriander
1 teaspoon ground turmeric

Drain and rinse the chickpeas. Place in a pan and cover with cold water. Bring to the boil, then drain and rinse again under cold water. Mix the ingredients for the spice mixture in a small bowl. Heat 2 tablespoons of oil in a large casserole and cook the onions gently for about 8 minutes until soft. Add the spice mixture and mix well. Add the chickpeas, cover and simmer for 1 hour. Place the chicken in the casserole and cover with more cold water. Bring to the boil, then cover and simmer for 30 minutes.

Put the couscous in a bowl with a pinch of salt and cover with boiling water. Leave to stand, stirring occasionally until all the water has been absorbed. Stir in the remaining oil, cinnamon and orange-flower water (if desired).

Add all the vegetables except the courgettes to the stew and stir well. To steam the couscous, put it in a colander and place over the stew and cover with a lid. Cook over a medium heat for about 30 minutes, until the steam starts to rise through the couscous.

Add the raisins and courgettes to the stew 15 minutes before the end of the cooking time and season with salt and pepper to taste.

Pile the couscous on a flat serving dish. Remove the chicken, chickpeas and vegetables from the cooking liquid with a slotted spoon and arrange over the couscous. Moisten with a few spoons of the liquid and serve the remainder separately. Garnish with the coriander leaves.

Salad of Fruits and Ginger

(Serves 6)

1 small pineapple

1 small Ogen melon

2 ripe Comice pears

juice of ½ lemon

50g drained stem ginger

90ml white wine

1 teaspoon sweetener

1 tablespoon liqueur (optional)

Heat the wine and sweetener together, add the liqueur (if desired) and allow to cool. Prepare the fruit and cut neatly into mouth-sized pieces. Dip the pear in the lemon juice to avoid discolouring. Chop the stem ginger. Mix the fruits and ginger together and pour over the wine. Cover and chill.

Normandy Sausages

(Serves 4)

8 pork sausages with herbs

2 tablespoons virgin olive oil

16 sage leaves

2 onions, sliced

225g seedless green grapes

150ml dry cider

1 teaspoon arrowroot

salt and freshly ground black pepper

Heat the oil in a frying pan and gently fry the sage leaves for a few minutes. Remove and put aside. Add the onions and cook until soft. Remove and put aside.

Cook the sausages in the same pan over a medium heat for about 10 minutes, turning occasionally until they are well browned on all sides. Return the onions and sage leaves to the pan, add the grapes and stir in the dry cider.

Mix the arrowroot with 1 tablespoon of water and add to the pan. Stir until thickened. Add salt and pepper to taste, cover and simmer for 5 minutes.

Fruit and Vegetable Curry

(Serves 4)

1 large onion, finely chopped
175g swede, diced
175g carrot, diced
175g parsnip, diced
2 tablespoons virgin oil
½ teaspoon chilli powder
½ teaspoon coriander powder
½ teaspoon turmeric
½ teaspoon cumin seeds
175g cauliflower, broken into florets
2 sharp green eating apples, peeled and chopped
15g butter
coriander leaves for garnish

Cook the root vegetables in the oil in a large pan over a medium heat for about 5 minutes. Add the spices and 285ml water and simmer for 15 minutes. Stir in the cauliflower. Cover and simmer for a further 20 minutes. Add the apple and simmer for a further 4 minutes. Garnish with the coriander.

Salmon in a Parcel

(Serves 4)

4 x 175g salmon steaks

5 teaspoons virgin olive oil

4 teaspoons balsamic vinegar

sprig of dill

salt and freshly ground black pepper

Cut 4 squares of greaseproof paper and 4 squares of foil large enough to enclose the steaks. Place the greaseproof squares on top of the foil. Brush the greaseproof paper with 1 teaspoon of the olive oil, then place the steaks on the top. Drizzle 1 teaspoon of oil and 1 teaspoon of balsamic vinegar on each steak, season well with salt and pepper, and top with a sprig of dill. Wrap the steaks carefully and cook at 220°C/gas mark 7 for about 8 minutes, when the fish should be just opaque.

Vegetable Rainbow

(Serves 4)

240g broad beans, unshelled
180g young carrots, diced
180g young white turnips
90g frozen peas
2 tablespoons herbs, freshly chopped
2 tablespoons low-fat mayonnaise
1 parsley sprig
salt and freshly ground black pepper

Cook the vegetables carefully so that they remain fairly crisp. Strain and season with salt and pepper, fold in the herbs and the mayonnaise. Garnish with the parsley.

Florida Cocktail

(Serves 1)

Arrange segments of orange and grapefruit alternately in a circle on a plate and garnish with chopped mint.

Oriental Combination Salad

(Serves 4–6)

225g packet of mixed salad leaves
2 oranges
4 canned water chestnuts, sliced
2 teaspoons sesame seeds
1 pear
2 ripe persimmons

DRESSING

1 ripe persimmon
1 tablespoon fruit vinegar
1 teaspoon sesame oil
1 teaspoon lemon juice
½ teaspoon soy sauce
salt and freshly ground black pepper

Peel the oranges, removing the pith and segment neatly. Cover the water chestnuts with water and keep cool. Toast the sesame seeds in a dry pan, being careful not to burn them, and put aside

To make the dressing, peel 1 persimmon and put in a blender together with ½ cup of water, the vinegar, sesame oil, lemon juice and soy sauce. Add salt and pepper to taste, and blend well. Keep cool. When ready to serve, slice the pear and the other persimmons.

Mix the salad with the dressing and arrange the fruit and water chestnuts on the top. Sprinkle with the toasted sesame seeds.

Smoked Chicken Salad

(Serves 4)
2 smoked, skinned and boneless chicken breasts
1 tablespoon virgin olive oil
350g salad spinach
175g button mushrooms, sliced
4 spring onions, sliced
1 large ripe avocado, peeled, stoned and diced
squeeze of lemon juice

DRESSING

1 garlic clove, crushed
4 tablespoons low-fat natural yogurt
juice of 1 orange
1½ teaspoons white wine vinegar
1 teaspoon Dijon mustard
½ teaspoon Tabasco sauce
2 tablespoons parsley, freshly chopped
freshly ground black pepper

Pre-heat the oven to 190°C/gas mark 5. Place the chicken breasts on an oiled baking tray and cook for 10 minutes on each side.

Wash and dry the spinach.

Combine all the ingredients for the dressing except the parsley, and mix well.

Coat the avocado well with the lemon juice.

When the chicken is cooked, cut into cubes and stir any juices into the dressing. While the chicken is still warm, mix with the avocado, salad spinach, button mushrooms and spring onions, and sprinkle with the parsley. Serve the dressing in a small jug.

Navarin of Lamb

(Serves 4)

450g neck fillet of lamb, cut into 50mm chunks
4 medium onions, quartered
4 medium carrots, halved crosswise
4 small turnips, halved
4 small potatoes
2 garlic cloves, crushed
570ml lamb stock
2 tablespoons tomato purée
bouquet garni
2 sprigs fresh rosemary
2 teaspoons arrowroot
salt and freshly ground black pepper
parsley for garnish

Place the lamb, onions, carrots, turnips, whole potatoes and the garlic in a casserole. Add the lamb stock, tomato purée, bouquet garni and rosemary sprigs, and bring to a simmer. Cover with a lid and cook for about 2¼ hours until the meat is tender.

Mix the arrowroot with 1 tablespoon of water and stir into the casserole. Cook until slightly thickened. Remove the bouquet garni and rosemary. Add salt and pepper to taste, and garnish with chopped parsley.

Prawn Stir-fry

(Serves 4)

225g peeled raw prawns

1 medium onion, thinly sliced

175g mangetout, topped and tailed

1 large ripe mango, peeled and neatly sliced

1 tablespoon sesame oil

2 teaspoons fresh ginger, grated

1 tablespoon dry sherry

1 tablespoon soy sauce

1 level teaspoon arrowroot

Heat the oil in a wok, and stir-fry the onions and ginger for 2 minutes until just tender. Add the mangetout and prawns and stir-fry for 1 minute, until the prawns turn pink.

Add the mango, sherry and soy sauce, and stir-fry for 1 minute. Mix the arrowroot with 1 tablespoon of water and stir into the mixture for 2 minutes until thickened.

Exotic Chicken with Spicy Fruits

(Serves 4)

4 x 275g skinless and fatless chicken quarters
285ml chicken stock
150ml orange juice
2 teaspoons paprika
2 teaspoons ground ginger
½ teaspoon ground cinnamon
¼ teaspoon ground allspice
250g packet ready-to-eat mixed dried fruit
salt and freshly ground black pepper

Pour the stock and the orange juice into a flameproof casserole, add the spices and stir well. Add the dried fruit and bring slowly to the boil, stirring. Add the chicken and add salt and pepper to taste. Baste the chicken well with the liquid.

Reduce the heat, cover the pan tightly and simmer very gently for about 30 minutes, stirring occasionally, until the chicken is tender. Adjust seasoning and serve.

Britney Spears has a punishing workout of 1,000 sit-ups every day and four 90-minute gym sessions a week!

Cameron Diaz enjoys surfing and martial arts to keep herself gorgeous. She works out using Wing Chun, a kind of Kung Fu, which strengthens the arms, shoulders and waist, but is particularly effective for those stubborn hips, bums and tums.

Roast Loin of Pork with Prunes

(Serves 6–8)

1.4kg loin of pork, boned and with rind and excess fat removed
12 ready-to-eat prunes
285ml white grape juice
285ml chicken stock
2 shallots, chopped
12 crushed juniper berries
3 tablespoons sloe gin (optional)
1 level tablespoon arrowroot

Using a sharp knife, make a large hole in the centre of the eye of the loin and press the prunes into it.

Put the pork in an ovenproof dish just large enough to hold the meat, pour over the juice and stock, then add the shallots and juniper berries. Pre-heat oven to 190°C/gas mark 5 and cook for about 1¼ hours or until the pork is tender. Remove the pork and let it stand for 5 minutes before carving.

Transfer the cooking juices to a pan and add the gin (if desired). Mix the arrowroot with 1 tablespoon of cold water and use to thicken the juices. Carve the meat and serve the sauce separately.

Pea and Ham Risotto

(Serves 4)

350g risotto rice

4 thin slices lean cooked ham, cut into thin strips

½ large onion, finely chopped

2 tablespoons virgin olive oil

15g butter

1.1 litres vegetable stock

150ml dry white wine

75g frozen peas

50g Parmesan cheese, freshly grated

salt and freshly ground black pepper

Heat the oil and butter in a large saucepan over a gentle heat and cook the onion for 5 minutes until soft. Mix in the rice and continue to cook over a moderate heat until the grains begin to burst. Meanwhile, heat the stock.

Stir the wine into the rice until it has been absorbed. Add 150ml of the hot stock, mix well and cook over a moderate heat until absorbed, stirring constantly.

Continue cooking for 20 minutes, adding the stock in 150ml quantities, until the rice is tender yet firm and the texture is creamy. Add the peas with the last measure of stock and add salt and pepper to taste. Fold in the ham and half of the Parmesan cheese. Divide between serving bowls and sprinkle with the remaining cheese.

Beef Bourguignon

(Serves 4)

450g chuck steak, cut into 40mm cubes
115g lean smoked bacon
1 large garlic clove, crushed
175g large button mushrooms
450g shallots
1 bouquet garni
450ml beef stock
285ml red Burgundy wine
2 teaspoons arrowroot
salt and freshly ground black pepper
parsley for garnish

Cut the rinds off the bacon and fry them gently in a flameproof casserole to release some of the fat. Discard the rinds and fry the bacon for 2 minutes on each side. Drain the bacon on kitchen paper and cut into small pieces.

Place the chuck steak in the casserole, together with the garlic, the mushrooms, shallots, bouquet garni, stock and wine. Add salt and pepper to taste.

Bring the casserole to a simmer, then cover and cook in the oven at 160°C/gas mark 3 for about 3 hours. Stir occasionally and check for tenderness.

Mix the arrowroot with 2 tablespoons water, stir into the casserole and simmer until thickened. Add the bacon, adjust the seasoning and garnish with the parsley.

Parsnip and Apple Soup

(Serves 6)

450g parsnips, roughly chopped
1 medium onion, finely chopped
2½ tablespoons virgin olive oil
250g Cox's apples, chopped
½ teaspoon ground nutmeg
850ml vegetable stock
285ml semi-skimmed milk
salt and freshly ground black pepper
parsley sprigs for garnish

Heat the oil in a large pan and cook the onion over a medium heat until transparent.

Stir the nutmeg into the onion and add the parsnips, apple and stock. Bring to the boil, then reduce the heat and simmer for about 20 minutes until the parsnips are tender. Allow to cool slightly.

Blend the soup in a liquidiser until smooth. Stir in the milk and reheat gently, adding salt and pepper to taste. Garnish with the parsley and serve.

Warm Scallop Salad

(Serves 6)

350g fresh or frozen scallops
salt
175g mangetout
1 oak-leaf lettuce
50g rocket
50mm fresh root ginger
2 tablespoons extra virgin olive oil
1 tablespoon light soy sauce
3 tablespoons dry sherry

Trim the mangetout and blanch in salted, boiling water for 2 minutes. Drain and refresh in cold water. Wash and dry the lettuce and the rocket leaves. Divide between 6 small plates, with the mangetout. Cover and chill until required.

Peel the ginger and slice it into very thin strips. Blanch the strips by plunging into boiling water for 30 seconds. Then put into ice-cold water, drain and pat dry. Mix the olive oil with the soy sauce. Cut large scallops into three, but leave small ones whole.

Pour the sherry into a small pan and bring to the boil. Add the scallops, cover with a lid and cook for 2 minutes or until the scallops are just cooked, shaking the pan continuously.

Remove the scallops from the pan and divide between the 6 plates. Scatter the strips of ginger over the scallops. Add 3 tablespoons of the liquid left in the pan to the soy sauce mixture. Shake well, pour the dressing over the salads and serve at once.

Spicy Kebabs with Cucumber Dip

(Serves 4)

700g lamb fillet, cut into bite-sized pieces

3 teaspoons fresh root ginger

3 tablespoons light soy sauce

3 tablespoons dark soy sauce

12 baby onions

DIP

½ cucumber, coarsely grated

1 garlic clove, crushed

2 teaspoons mint, freshly chopped

150ml natural yogurt

salt and freshly ground black pepper

Place the lamb in a large bowl. Peel and grate the ginger. Combine the ginger and the two soy sauces and add to the lamb, mixing well. Leave to marinate for about 12 hours.

To make the dip, combine the cucumber, garlic, mint, yogurt, and salt and pepper to taste. Cover and store in the refrigerator until required.

Cook the onions whole in boiling water for 5 minutes, then drain and remove the skins.

Pre-heat the grill. Thread the lamb pieces and onions alternately on to 4 kebab sticks and grill, turning and basting frequently, for about 15 minutes. Serve with the dip.

Goldie Hawn

WILD BEAUTY Goldie Hawn has a figure, even in her sixties, that would be the envy of a teenager. Tall, slim, youthful, she is what all women would like to be as they grow older. Goldie's secret lies not just in the workouts she does in her specially installed private gymnasium, but also in the dieting regime she lays down for herself.

Goldie has been known to follow a strict wheat-free, sugar-free and dairy-free diet, one of the most consistent features of which is what she calls 'green juice' – a fresh vegetable juice made from celery, kale, parsley and green peppers. But this isn't the only juice you can drink if you fancy a day of detox. In fact, whole books have been written on the subject. Here are just a few delicious juices you can try – they almost feel like a meal in a glass, they are fantastically low-fat and they taste great.

To make these juices you will need a good-quality juicer: it's a purchase you'll never regret and it can be the dieter's best friend. Always remember that, unless you are used to drinking large quantities of fresh juice, it is recommended that to start with you consume a maximum of three 240ml portions a day.

Simply pass the items listed in the following recipes through a juicer, only peeling or coring if the recipe says so:

Slimmer's Juice 1

Apples are very effective for breaking down fatty foods.

2 apples
2 kiwi fruit
2 pears
1 stick of celery

Slimmer's Juice 2

Watercress was used in the eighteenth century as a cure for hangovers, but as you're a successful slimmer you won't be drinking alcohol to excess.

2 apples
2 carrots, topped and tailed
2 tomatoes
a bunch of watercress
a handful of spinach

Slimmer's Juice 3

4 satsumas, peeled
2 carrots, topped and tailed
1 large apple
1 large parsnip

FAMOUS PEOPLE DON'T GET FAT

Former Eastender *Nathalie Cassidy* always has some healthy home-made soup in the fridge for when she comes home late at night, to avoid the temptation to snack on convenience foods.

Liz Hurley

LIZ'S SLIMMING regime can be summed up with one little word – watercress! She makes herself a delicious watercress soup, and she says of it: 'It's fatless, low-calorie, full of vitamins and iron and delicious enough to serve at a dinner party. I drink at least six cups a day when eager to lose a few pounds.'

Six cups! It would need to be a delicious soup indeed in order to keep that up. But guess what – it is! What's more, there is a fantastic week-long diet you can follow that centres around this amazing soup. By following the watercress soup diet, you can lose up to 4.5kg in seven days – *and never feel hungry*. As long as you follow the diet strictly, you can eat as much as you want of certain foods, including meat, fish, vegetables and fruit. It's fantastic.

So how do you go about it? Well, first you need to learn how to make watercress soup:

Watercress Soup

1 small onion, finely chopped
1.5 litres light chicken stock or water
2 small potatoes, diced
3 large bunches of watercress, with stems removed
salt and pepper

Sweat the onion in 2–3 tablespoons of chicken stock or water. Add the potatoes, stock, salt and pepper, bring to the boil and simmer until the potatoes are soft. Add the watercress and stir for 3 minutes. Remove from the heat, allow to cool slightly and blend in a liquidiser.

Pour the soup into a metal bowl and put this in a sink full of ice-cold water. This will keep the lovely green colour of the soup. The soup is delicious drunk either hot or cold.

Once you've done that, all you need to know is what you can eat on each of the seven days of the watercress soup diet:

DAY 1

Unlimited watercress soup

Unlimited fruit from the fruit list

250ml skimmed milk or fat-free yogurt

DAY 2

Unlimited watercress soup

Unlimited vegetables from the vegetable list

1 jacket potato

250ml skimmed milk or fat-free yogurt

DAY 3

Unlimited watercress soup

Unlimited fruit from the fruit list

Unlimited vegetables from the vegetable list

250ml skimmed milk or fat-free yogurt

DAY 4

Unlimited watercress soup

5 bananas

8 x 250ml portions skimmed milk (one of which can be replaced with 250ml fat-free yogurt)

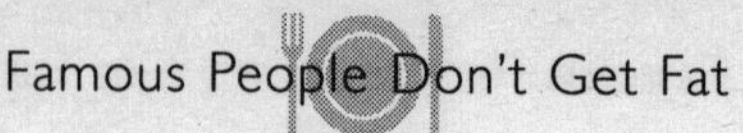

DAY 5

Unlimited watercress soup
Unlimited white fish
Unlimited skinless, lean chicken
6 medium tomatoes or 1 can
250ml skimmed milk or fat-free yogurt

DAY 6

Unlimited watercress soup
Unlimited white fish
Unlimited skinless, lean chicken
Unlimited vegetables from the vegetable list
Unlimited tomatoes
250ml skimmed milk or fat-free yogurt

DAY 7

Unlimited watercress soup
Unlimited fruit from the fruit list
Unlimited vegetables from the vegetable list
250ml skimmed milk or fat-free yogurt

The Watercress Soup Diet Fruit List

Apples
Apricots
Blackberries
Blueberries
Cherries
Grapefruit
Grapes
Kiwi fruit
Lemons
Melons
Nectarines
Oranges
Peaches
Pineapples
Plums
Raspberries
Strawberries
Tangerines

The Watercress Soup Diet Vegetable List

Artichokes
Asparagus
Aubergines
Beans
Beetroot
Broccoli
Brussels sprouts
Cabbages
Carrots
Cauliflowers
Celery
Courgettes
Cucumbers
Lettuces
Mushrooms
Onions
Parsley
Peppers
Radishes
Spinach
Turnips
Watercress

There are a few simple rules you need to follow:

- Don't skip foods – everything is there for a reason, so make sure you eat what's on the list so that you don't miss out on essential nutrients.

- Don't overeat. Have as much as you need to stop feeling hungry and no more.

- On each day, you can eat *either* milk or yogurt. The only day you are allowed to mix them is Day 4.

- You can use flavourings and condiments but only as long as they contain less than 25 calories per teaspoon.

- This is a very intensive weight-loss programme, and it should be used for no more than one week at a time.

And that's it. Follow this diet and get a few steps closer to that Liz Hurley gorgeousness!

Day-time TV queen *Fern Briton* owes her healthy complexion to a balanced diet prepared by celebrity chef husband Phil Vickery – plenty of fruit and vegetables help improve skin tone and texture.

Angelina Jolie

Wow! Fit, lean, perfectly toned – that's Angelina Jolie in *Tomb Raider*, and if she looked great before, she looks fantastic now.

To get that mega-fit body, Angelina follows a high-carbohydrate, high-protein, low-fat diet, coupled with an intensive exercise regime. The carbohydrates provide the energy for the exercise, and the protein increases the muscle tissue. She also tries to eat five small meals regularly throughout the day.

Try the diets below to get a Lara Croft figure for yourself. But remember, these recipes are only suitable if you are exercising vigorously. As well as the five small meals a day, you can have two pieces of fruit, 250ml of skimmed milk and unlimited water – and remember to drink plenty of water – but even more if you're exercising a lot.

MENU 1

7 AM

50g Shredded Wheat with 200ml skimmed milk

10 AM

1 banana mashed and topped with 60g fresh strawberries

1 Scotch pancake topped with 1 poached egg

1 PM

150g grilled salmon, 50g peas, watercress

4 PM

33g muesli bar

150g orange juice

7 PM

130g chicken breast cooked in a parcel with lemon juice and sliced tomatoes

100g baked potato

200g rice pudding with 60g fresh blackcurrants

MENU 2

7 AM

60g muesli served with 60g grated apple and 200ml skimmed milk

10 AM

70g toasted bagel topped with 40g low-fat cottage cheese with mixed herbs and topped with 65g grilled tomato

1 PM

125g grilled plaice fillets
190g pasta in tomato sauce
½ grapefruit

4 PM

1 small scone with low-fat spread and 1 teaspoon honey

7 PM

140g grilled lean steak
175g new potatoes
Large green salad
125g fresh fruit salad

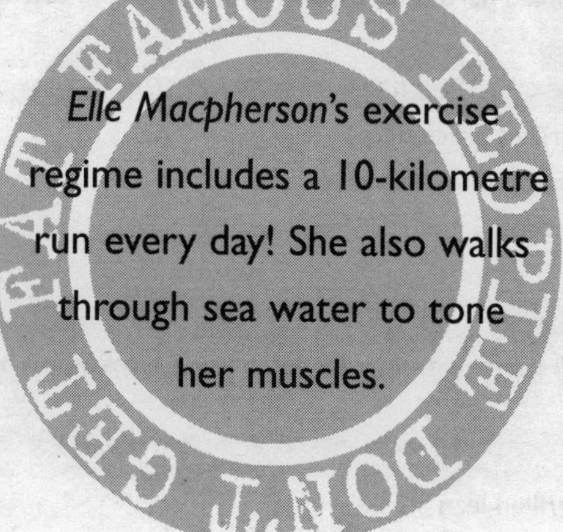

Elle Macpherson's exercise regime includes a 10-kilometre run every day! She also walks through sea water to tone her muscles.

FAMOUS PEOPLE DON'T GET FAT

Robbie Williams keeps the girls screaming over his pop-star good looks by regular kick-boxing sessions and Sunday morning football matches.

MENU 3

7 AM

125g cooked porridge with 200ml skimmed milk
125g banana

10 AM

1 slice (25g) wholemeal bread topped with 75g sardines in spring water
75g grapes

1 PM

75g chicken, 75g roast potatoes (using spray oil), 175g steamed broccoli
75g canned tangerines

4 PM

Crackers with 115g cream cheese

7 PM

125g halibut with 200g baked potato
Mixed salad of cherry tomatoes, watercress and mushrooms tossed in a low-fat dressing

MENU 4

7 AM

80g banana, 60g raspberries, 350ml skimmed milk blended into a smoothie

10 AM

125g baked beans on 50g wholemeal bread
1 apple

1 PM

125g prawns served with 50g savoury rice (mix with chopped mixed herbs, lemon juice and sprinkle liberally with chopped chives)
Mixed salad
125g strawberries

4 PM

2 digestive biscuits
25g cheese
1 pear

7 PM

75g grilled lean pork chop
2 grilled tomatoes
125g cauliflower
200g rice pudding with 1 teaspoon honey

MENU 5

7 AM

50g Weetabix served with 200ml skimmed milk

10 AM

2-egg omelette cooked with 50g cheese

1 grilled tomato

25g wholemeal toast

1 PM

125g steamed trout served with 75g (uncooked weight) spaghetti with pesto and green salad

Baked apple with 25g raisins

4 PM

33g muesli bar

small banana

7 PM

125g boiled gammon with 50g parsley sauce

25g peas, 25g sweetcorn, 25g carrots, 50g new potatoes

2 peaches poached with sweetener and served with 1 tablespoon low-fat crème fraîche

Jordan

HER WAISTLINE may not be the part of her anatomy for which über-model Katie Price – known to almost everyone as Jordan – is most renowned, but you don't become one of the world's most famous celebrity models without maintaining a figure to die for. And while it may not be the case that she avoids some of the excesses of the celebrity lifestyle, there can be no doubt that she is scrupulous in watching what she eats so that she continues to look fabulous.

Jordan has lately revealed that she owes her amazing figure to what she calls the Apple and Celery Diet. It's not as odd as it sounds – both ingredients are healthy and low in fat, and it is well known that an eating plan based around fruit and vegetables is good both for your health and for your waistline. In the pages that follow, you will find a number of lunch and dinner suggestions that form part of the Apple and Celery Diet. They're all delicious, and they might just change the way you think about your food!

Just For One

(Serves 1)

50g cottage cheese
2 sticks celery
90g chopped apple
25g walnuts
lettuce
lemon juice

Mix together the cottage cheese, celery, apple and walnuts. Serve on the salad leaves dressed with lemon juice.

Healthy Salad

(Serves 1)

½ small red onion, chopped
90g apple or pear, chopped
2 sticks of celery, chopped
2 inch piece of cucumber, chopped
4 medium mushrooms, chopped
25g raisins
½ garlic clove, crushed
250ml low-fat natural yoghurt
watercress to serve

Mix together all the ingredients, then serve on a bed of watercress.

Red Cabbage, Apple and Celery Casserole

(Serves 6)

450g red cabbage, sliced very thinly
2 apples, peeled and roughly chopped
2 medium onions, peeled and roughly chopped
4 sticks celery, roughly chopped
2 rashers bacon, chopped
2 teaspoons caraway seeds
2 teaspoons horseradish
300ml plain yoghurt
salt and freshly ground black pepper

Preheat the oven to 160°C/gas mark 3.

Mix the first six ingredients in a bowl. Combine the horseradish with the yoghurt, season lightly and spoon over the vegetables. Mix the whole lot together and turn into an ovenproof casserole. Bake for 45 minutes, removing the dish once or twice to stir. The cabbage should still be crisp at the end of the cooking. Serve the dish hot with rye bread or plain boiled potatoes.

Celery and Water Chestnut Casserole

(Serves 4)

50g low-fat margarine

1 medium head celery, cleaned and diced

1 medium onion, finely chopped

225g button mushrooms with their stems, wiped and halved

1 x 400g tin water chestnuts, halved, with their liquid

25g flour

150ml dry white wine or cider

100g herb cream cheese

90ml crème fraîche

50g flaked almonds

50g brown breadcrumbs

salt and freshly ground black pepper

Melt the margarine in a heavy-based pan and gently sweat the celery and onion for about 15 minutes until they begin to soften. Add the mushrooms and cook for a couple of minutes, then add the water chestnuts, reserving their liquid. Sift in the flour, stir the mixture well and cook for a couple of minutes. Gradually add the liquid from the water chestnuts, the wine and the cheese. Slowly bring back to the boil and cook for a couple of minutes until the sauce thickens. Add the crème fraîche and the flaked almonds and season to taste.

Spoon the mixture into a serving dish, sprinkle the breadcrumbs over the top and grill for a couple of minutes until crisp.

Apple, Celery and Parsnip Soup

(Serves 6)

1 medium onion, finely chopped
2 sticks celery, chopped
2 tablespoons olive oil
a good grinding of nutmeg
450g parsnips, peeled and roughly chopped
250g Cox's apples, peeled, cored and roughly chopped
225ml semi-skimmed milk
850ml vegetable stock
salt and freshly ground black pepper
chopped parsley to garnish

Soften the onions and the celery in the oil. Stir in the nutmeg and add the parsnips, apple, milk and stock. Bring to the boil, then reduce the heat and simmer for about 20 minutes until the parsnips are tender. Allow to cool then pour into a food processor and blend until smooth. Garnish with the parsley.

Mediterranean Salad

(Serves 1)

½ small little gem lettuce, washed and torn into pieces
a handful of watercress
1 medium tomato, sliced
2 inches cucumber, sliced
½ red pepper, finely sliced
1 stick celery, finely sliced
25g green beans
1 small hard-boiled egg
25g tuna (in brine)
1 tablespoon lemon juice
1 tablespoon olive oil
½ crisp apple, chopped

Cover the plate with the lettuce and watercress, then lay the tomato, cucumber, pepper and celery on top. Cook the beans until al dente. Flake the tuna. Slice the egg and add to the plate together with the warm beans and tuna.

Mix the lemon juice and olive oil with the apple and spoon over the top.

Herrings and Apple in Oatmeal

(Serves 6)

6 herrings, cleaned, boned and cut in half (ask your fishmonger to do this)

6 tablespoons porridge oats

4 tablespoons good wholegrain mustard

50g butter

2 tablespoons vegetable oil

4 crisp eating apples, peeled, cored and cut into wedges

celery curls to garnish

Dry the herrings, then coat them on both sides in a paste made by combining the oats and the mustard. Melt 25g of the butter and the oil together and fry the herrings gently on both sides until just cooked. Keep warm.

Wipe out the pan. Add the remaining butter and gently cook the apples, keeping them quite crisp. Serve them with the fish and garnish the dish with the celery curls.

Low-fat Chicken Dinner

(Serves 6)

12 small skinless chicken thighs

3 large leeks, cleaned and roughly sliced

3 sticks celery, sliced

3 carrots, sliced

2 tablespoons chopped fresh mixed herbs (or use 2 teaspoons dried)

400ml light chicken stock

280ml dry white wine.

200g tin tomatoes

6 tablespoons wholemeal pasta shapes

salt and freshly ground black pepper

Put the chicken with the vegetables, herbs and seasoning into a large pot and pour in the liquid. Cover the pan, bring to the boil and simmer for 25 minutes. Now add the tomatoes and the pasta. Bring to the boil again and simmer for about 20 minutes. Ensure the chicken is thoroughly cooked. You can serve this dish like an Irish stew – a small bowl of soup first, followed by the chicken and vegetables.

Grey Mullet with Plum and Chilli Sauce served with an Apple and Celery Salad

(Serves 6)

25g butter

1 small onion, finely chopped

75g fresh or frozen (not tinned) gooseberries

3 red plums

1 whole red chilli, seeded and finely chopped

6 grey mullet, filleted

slices of lemon

a little white wine and water mixed

DRESSING

1 bag rocket

2 sharp Granny Smith apples, peeled and chopped

3 sticks of celery

2 tablespoons olive oil

1 tablespoon fresh lemon juice

Preheat the oven to 180°C/gas mark 4.

Melt the butter in a small pan and gently cook the onion, gooseberries, plums and chopped chilli for 10 to 15 minutes until they are totally mushy. Purée them in a food processor and taste. If the sauce is too sour for your taste, add a little sweetener, but not too much.

Lay the fillets in an ovenproof dish, surround with the lemon slices and just cover with the wine and water. Cover and bake for about 15 minutes until just done. Mix the salad ingredients together and toss in the oil and lemon juice, seasoning with a little salt and freshly ground pepper. Serve the mullet, sharing the salad between the six plates.

Casserole of Pheasant with Apples and Celery

(Serves 2)

25g butter

1 pheasant

1 small onion, finely chopped

55g bacon lardons

1 stick celery, roughly chopped

2 sprigs sage

1 Granny Smith apple, peeled, cored and cut into chunks

250ml dry cider

145ml chicken stock

2 Cox's apples, peeled and cored

15g melted butter

½ tablespoon light brown sugar

fresh spinach to serve

salt and freshly ground black pepper

Preheat oven to 190°C/gas mark 5.

Melt the butter in non-stick, flameproof casserole. Season the pheasant, place it in the pot on top of the stove and brown it all over. Remove from the pan and set aside.

Add the onion, bacon, celery and sage to the pot and cook over a medium heat until the onion is soft and translucent and the bacon is crispy. Pour off any excess fat.

Return the pheasant to the pot and sprinkle over the Granny Smith apple. Add 125ml of the cider and the chicken stock. Bring to a gentle simmer and place in the oven for about 20 minutes.

Place the apples on a baking tray that has been brushed with a little butter and sprinkle with the sugar. Place in the oven and bake for about 30 minutes.

Remove the pheasant and place on a chopping board. Remove the thighs and breasts and set aside to keep warm. Chop the carcass into two pieces and place back into the pot with the other 125ml cider. Bring to the boil and simmer gently for 5 minutes.

Strain the sauce into a bowl through a sieve. Pour the strained stock back into the pot and reduce by half. Add the cream and simmer for a few minutes. Put the pheasant back into the sauce so that each piece is well coated. Serve on a bed of lightly cooked spinach.

Prawn Pilaff

(Serves 4)

4 tablespoons olive oil

1 small onion, peeled and finely chopped

1 small red pepper, finely chopped

1 stick celery, veins removed with a vegetable peeler and finely chopped

1 garlic clove, finely chopped

4 heaped tablespoons long-grain patna rice

½ teaspoon ground allspice

½ teaspoon cumin seeds

1 heaped teaspoon dried mint or basil

100g king prawns, peeled

2 tablespoons currants

1 small eating apple, peeled and chopped

juice of 1 large or 2 small lemons

2 tablespoons finely chopped parsley

salt and freshly ground black pepper

Heat the oil in a large, flat pan and gently cook the onion, peppers celery and garlic until they are soft but not browned. Add the rice, spices and herbs and stir together for a few minutes. Now add enough water to cover the rice. Bring the mixture to the boil and simmer with the pan uncovered for 10–15 minutes or until the rice is just cooked but not mushy. You may have to add a little more water if it dries up too fast. Add the prawns, currants, apple and a generous sprinkling of salt. Warm through for a couple of minutes, add the lemon juice and parsley and adjust the seasoning to taste. This may be served warm or cold.

FAMOUS PEOPLE DON'T GET FAT

Singing sensation *Beyoncé* believes the secret to her slimming success is everything in moderation: 'If I want something naughty, then I just have a little bite of it!'

Ashley Judd

SVELTE ASHLEY Judd grew up in the American south, where the food can hardly be said to be helpful to the dieter – fried chicken, pies and cakes were the staples. So what are Ashley's tips for staying slim?

Every morning when she wakes up she has a cup of hot water and lemon – a great way to flush out your system and perk you up. Aside from that, she uses a lot of herbs in her cooking to make her low-fat dishes more interesting. Both fresh and dried herbs are brilliant fat-free flavourings which can be used in thousands of different ways. Here are a few delicious, low-fat, low-carb recipes which have been livened up with herbs:

Braised Celery Hearts

(Serves 6)

Celery is the all-year-round edible herb. Every part of this marvellous herb is usable: root, stalk, leaf and seed.

3 celery hearts, thoroughly washed and cut in half lengthwise
1 onion, chopped
1 bay leaf
1 beef stock cube
25g butter
25g flour
Marmite (optional)
salt

Place the celery hearts in a saucepan with 425ml of water, a little salt, the onion and the bay leaf. Bring to the boil, then remove the celery and onion from water and cool. Place in a lightly buttered shallow baking dish

Make a roux from the butter and flour and stir in the cooking water gradually to make a smooth sauce. Taste for flavour and add a little Marmite if necessary.

Pour the thin brown sauce over the celery, which is ready for the oven, now or later to suit your convenience. Bake at 200°C/gas mark 6 for about 45 minutes. This dish is delicious by itself, or served with some lightly grilled chicken and a side salad.

Drinks Party Canapé

To make a drinks party canapé using celery, trim as many celery sticks as you need of coarse strings (best done with a vegetable peeler). Fill the cavity with cottage cheese mixed with finely chopped chives and sprinkle with celery seeds. Cut into 4cm lengths and serve on a tray, garnished with watercress.

Dill-icious Cabbage Salad

(Serves 8)

1 large cabbage, finely shredded
1 cup celery, diced
50g parsley, chopped
100g low-fat crème fraîche or fromage frais
1 tablespoon onion, chopped
1 teaspoon dill seed
1 green pepper, thinly sliced
½ teaspoon salt
freshly ground black pepper

Combine all the ingredients, except the green pepper, in the order given. Toss lightly and decorate with green pepper.

You could serve this dish with a lightly steamed cutlet of salmon with the juice and zest of ½ lemon. Place the fish on a portion of the cabbage salad.

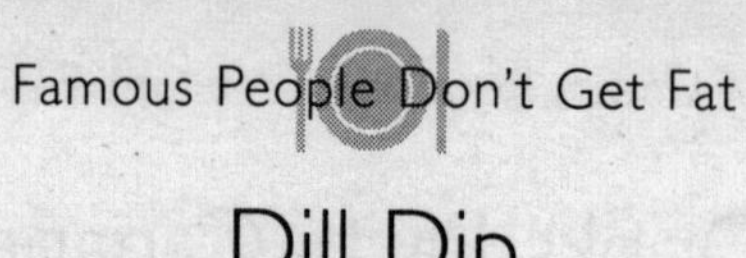

Dill Dip

150ml vinaigrette dressing
150ml very low-fat crème fraîche
1 tablespoon minced onion
1 tablespoon parsley, chopped
1 tablespoon dill seed or chopped dill leaves
1 teaspoon salt

Mix in the order given and serve with assorted vegetable sticks: carrot, celery, cucumber, cauliflower florets or peppers.

Veal Scallopine

(Serves 6)

900g veal cutlets
seasoned flour
25g butter
1 tablespoon vegetable oil
225 fresh mushrooms, sliced
200ml dry white wine
1 large onion, sliced
2 teaspoons sweetener
1 parsley sprig
¼ teaspoon dried rosemary
¼ teaspoon marjoram
¼ teaspoon peppercorns

Put the wine, onion, sweetener, parsley, herbs and peppercorns in a pan and bring to the boil. Simmer gently for 5 minutes, then leave to get cold.

Coat the cutlets lightly in seasoned flour. Brown them quickly in the butter and oil and dab well with kitchen paper. Put in a flameproof casserole and top with the mushrooms.

Pass the wine mixture through a sieve and pour over the meat and mushrooms. Cover tightly and simmer until meat is tender.

Serve with a portion of green vegetables and some carrots flavoured with lemon juice and chopped chives.

Baked Summer Marrow with Sage

(Serves 4)

1 ripe, unpeeled marrow

1 onion, chopped

a handful of fresh sage, chopped

25–50g butter (according to size of marrow)

salt and freshly ground black pepper

Cut the marrow into thin slices and arrange these in a buttered baking dish. Scatter the onion over the marrow. Sprinkle with sage, salt and pepper, and dot with the butter. Bake, uncovered, in pre-heated oven at 180°C/gas mark 4 until the marrow is tender.

Tarragon Tomatoes

(Serves 6–8)

5 large tomatoes, halved

175g low-fat cheese, grated

110g breadcrumbs

2 teaspoons tarragon, freshly chopped

½ teaspoon salt

freshly ground black pepper

Arrange the tomatoes in a lightly greased shallow baking dish that holds them snugly. Mix the cheese, breadcrumbs, tarragon, salt and pepper, and sprinkle over the tomatoes. Bake, uncovered, in a pre-heated oven at 190°C/gas mark 5 for about 30 minutes.

David Beckham keeps his fantastic footballer's figure in fine fettle by ditching the regular three meals a day in favour of six smaller snacks taken at regular intervals. That plus gruelling training sessions and 90-minute matches, of course.

Lisa Kudrow

YOU DON'T get a leading role in a show as popular as *Friends* if you don't look as good as you possibly can; and yet Lisa Kudrow's dieting techniques, like her character in the hit TV series, are a little kooky!

Lisa claims to have a voice inside her head which tells her when to stop eating. But perhaps this isn't as odd as it sounds. Most of us know when we are overindulging, and the trick of achieving a successful, life-long diet plan is to be in touch with your body and to know what you need and what you don't need. The little voice in Lisa's head is her way of being honest with herself about her dietary requirements, which should be the ultimate aim of every dieter.

Lisa does not limit herself to particular foods, but she does eat only certain sweets and chocolate. If you are a choc addict, then you would do well to do the same, and to be aware of the number of calories in each of the sweets you like – you will find that some are very much more calorific than others. Here is a list of some of the most popular sweets and their calories to help you on your way:

CALORIES PER 30G

Aero	150
After Eight	122
Bounty	135
Fry's Chocolate Creams	130
Fruit and Nut	145
Wholenut	185
Cadbury's Old Jamaica	130
Crunchie	145
Cadbury's Fudge	120
KitKat	145
Revels	135
Topic	135
Rolo	130
Fruit Gums	70

Fruit Pastilles	100
Jelly Babies	95
Liquorice All-Sorts	105
Smarties	130
Sweet Cigarettes	115
Maltesers	150
Mars Bar	130
Matchmakers	140
Milky Way	125
Minstrels	144
Glacier Mints	110
Opal Fruits	115
Peppermints	110
Polo Mints	115
Fry's Turkish Delight	110
Twix	145

Naomi Campbell likes to get active with a bit of boxercise to keep that supermodel body in shape. Her regular boxing classes go hand in hand with a diet that avoids wheat because she believes it encourages cellulite and water retention.

Nigel Lawson

LET'S FACE it, the former Chancellor of the Exchequer had the room to lose a little weight when he was in power. But he beat his critics when, after finding he could not stand up unaided following a fall while skiing, he set about losing an amazing 36kg in just 10 months.

Nigel followed this up by publishing his own book of dieting secrets, among them cutting out dairy products and other fatty foods and, interestingly, replacing alcoholic drinks with fizzy diet drinks. This is a very good idea, as alcohol is notoriously calorific, and although you shouldn't begrudge yourself the occasional glass of wine, you really should try to keep your consumption very moderate.

So what are you going to drink instead? Water's fine, and good for you, but sometimes you want something a bit more interesting, and you can only drink so much Diet Coke! Here's a list of a few ideas for alcohol substitutes – not all of them are right for all occasions, but they should help you cut down on your booze intake, and so improve your figure.

FRUIT AND HERBAL TEAS

Healthy, calming and restorative, fruit and herbal teas are a natural, fat-free drink that you can enjoy at any time. Buy them as teabags, or even make your own. (See pages 2-3 for information on herbal teas.)

SMOOTHIES

A super-food for slimmers and non-slimmers alike. Most supermarkets stock good fresh smoothies, or see pages 80-1 for ideas on how to make your own – it's very easy. Next time you feel like an aperitif, why not try a smoothie – they're far more delicious than a gin and tonic.

JUICE

We all know how delicious freshly squeezed orange juice is, but invest in a good-quality juicer and a whole new world of delicious, healthy juices will be open to you. (See pages 161 for more ideas.)

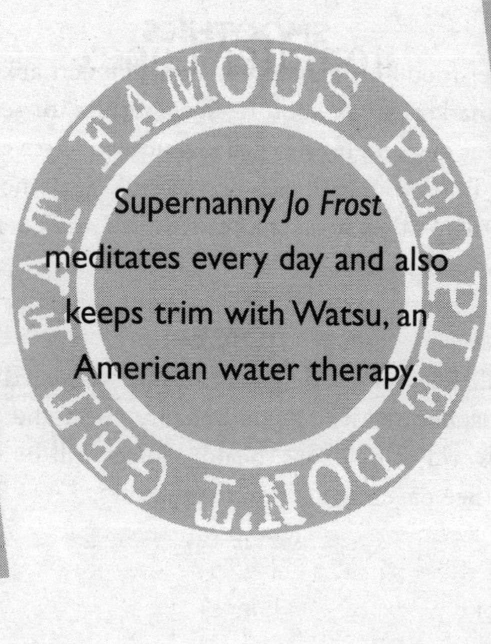

Supernanny *Jo Frost* meditates every day and also keeps trim with Watsu, an American water therapy.

Jennifer Lopez

THEY JUST don't come much sexier or more glamorous than Jennifer Lopez. Whether she has her singing or her acting hat on she always manages to look nothing less than stunning. Jennifer's secret is to eat healthily, but just a little and often. She eats eight 'mini-meals' a day to keep her energy level constantly high – and of course to keep hunger at bay.

A 'little-and-often' meal plan might look something like this – you can alter the timings to fit in with your own schedule, but try to keep your meals spaced at regular intervals to reap the full benefit of this regime:

DIET 1

8 am – small bowl cereal with skimmed milk
10 am – 1 banana
12 pm – 2 sardines in brine on 1 slice toast
2 pm – 2 satsumas
4 pm – 1 scone with cottage cheese
6 pm – 1 small jacket potato with low-fat spread
8 pm – 50g skinless chicken with a large mixed salad
10 pm – a mug of hot skimmed milk with 1 digestive biscuit

DIET 2

8 am – 1 boiled egg and 1 slice toast
10 am – 1 apple with 25g low-fat cheese
12 pm – 50g white fish and some steamed broccoli
2 pm – 12 grapes and 1 crispbread
4 pm – 1 slice wholemeal bread with honey
6 pm – 1 small portion Ratatouille (see page 135)
8 pm – 50g grilled lean fillet steak and 2 grilled tomatoes
10 pm – small bowl cereal with skimmed milk

DIET 3

8 am – 25g porridge oats with skimmed milk
10 am – 2 crispbread with cottage cheese
12 pm – 1 small can reduced-calorie baked beans with 1 slice (25g) toast
2 pm – 100g fruit salad
4 pm – 1 small pancake with lemon juice and sweetener
6 pm – bowl Watercress Soup (see pages 129 or 164)
8 pm – 1-egg omelette on a bed of spinach
10 pm – 25g lean ham on 1 slice (25g) bread and a mug of hot skimmed milk

To tone those A-list muscles, J-Lo practises a martial art used by the Israeli army called Krav Maga – it's not only a fantastic workout, but also a brilliant method of self-defence. If you want to try Krav Maga yourself, you can get more information from www.krav-maga.org.uk or by calling 07961 090 218. And J-Lo isn't the only celeb to practise Krav Maga – Tom Cruise is a fan too.

Kate Winslet lost an amazing 25kg by following the 'facial analysis diet'. Different-shaped faces require different dieting regimes. Sounds crazy? Well, if it worked for Kate, perhaps it can work for you too…

Sophie Loren

YEARS AFTER her heyday, this star of the silver screen still manages to look amazing. But then she does follow a very strict regime of what she can and can't eat. So what's in and what's out for Sophia Loren?

IN	OUT
Pasta	Crisps
Cheese	Cigarettes
Fruit and Vegetables	Alcohol

All standard stuff, apart from the pasta! But Sophia's Italian heritage could hardly allow her to cut the pasta from her diet, and there's no reason why you should have to either – in moderation. Here are some great, fairly dieting-friendly pasta meals for you to try:

Fusilli with Anchovies and Olives

(Serves 4)

It's best to make this with salted anchovies, or anchovies in brine, as they contain less fat than those in olive oil. To be authentically Italian you would sprinkle this dish with Parmesan cheese, but why not try any low-fat hard cheese as a substitute, or miss it out altogether? It will still be delicious.

375g dried fusilli
1 teaspoon vegetable oil
4 anchovy fillets, chopped
1 tablespoon tomato purée
12 pitted black olives, chopped
a small bunch of basil leaves
black pepper

Cook the pasta according to the instructions on the packet. Drain and put aside.

Heat the oil in a large saucepan. Add the anchovies, tomato purée and olives and stir until the mixture is hot. Season with black pepper.

Add the drained pasta to the pan and stir well so that all the pasta is coated. Tear up the basil leaves, add to the pasta, and serve immediately.

Linguini with Easy Tomato Sauce

(Serves 2)

You can make this with fresh tomatoes – you will need to peel them first by placing them in boiling water for a couple of minutes and then just slipping off the skins. But canned tomatoes are often more flavoursome for recipes like this.

200g dried linguini
1 400g can tomatoes
1 teaspoon olive oil
1 small onion, chopped
1 garlic clove, chopped
1 teaspoon dried basil or oregano
black pepper

Heat the oil in a saucepan and then gently soften the onions, being careful not to let them go brown. Add the tomatoes, herbs and pepper, stir, cover and simmer very gently for 10–15 minutes.

Cook the linguini in plenty of boiling water according to the instructions on the packet. Drain, then coat well with the tomato sauce. Season with a little more black pepper if you like, and serve immediately.

Elle Macpherson

TOP MODEL Elle Macpherson wasn't always so beautiful – she admits that as a teenager she was 'gawky and gangly'. But she knows you don't become one of the world's most beautiful women – with a nickname like 'The Body' – without carefully watching what you eat as well as exercising sensibly. This is why she does 500 – yes, 500! – stomach crunches every day.

She has also established a dieting regime which allows her to eat only twice a day – a healthy breakfast and then either lunch or dinner. It's important to eat a well-balanced diet if you are going to do this, and the plans that follow are created with this in mind. The great thing about this diet is that, as you are eating only twice a day, you can treat yourself a bit when you do eat – you'll see that some of the recipes that follow include goat's cheese or even a little cream. As long as you are eating sensibly and in moderation, you'll lose weight without too much trouble at all.

If you're at work during the day and decide you want to eat at lunchtime, that means preparing some good healthy food in advance to take to work with you. And if you want to eat in the evening, you need something that is slimming, nutritious and quick to prepare. Also, as you are going to eat only twice a day, your meals need to be reasonably substantial – just because you are on a diet doesn't mean you have to feel deprived! Here are a few ideas for both lunchtime and evening slimming. First there is a suggested menu plan, followed by all the recipes you will need. And remember, you can eat lunch or dinner – but not both – and only one portion of each dish!

MENU 1

BREAKFAST

50g porridge with skimmed milk

6 pitted prunes

1 slice toast with Marmite

Tea or coffee

LUNCH

Three Bean Pâté served with 1 small pitta bread and crudities (such as radishes, cauliflower florets, celery and carrot batons)

100g unsweetened fresh fruit salad and 1 small fat-free yogurt

or

DINNER

50g potato, mashed with a little low-fat crème fraîche

75g broccoli

100g unsweetened fresh fruit salad and 1 small fat-free yogurt

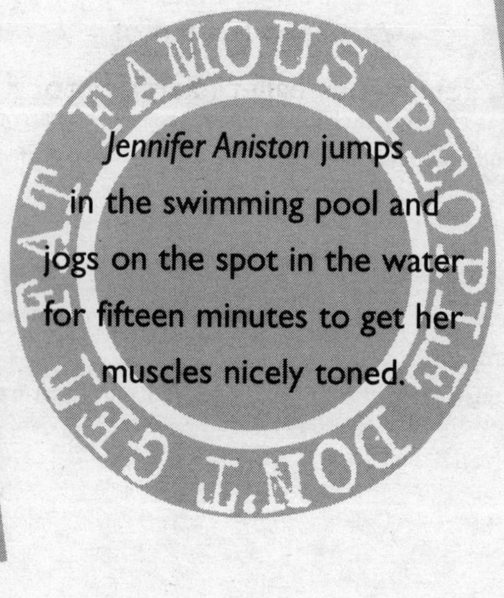

Jennifer Aniston jumps in the swimming pool and jogs on the spot in the water for fifteen minutes to get her muscles nicely toned.

Madonna is a fan of strenuous ballet exercises to keep in trim – and she's not the only celebrity to practise her pirouettes in order to stay slim – *Cameron Diaz* and *Gwyneth Paltrow* are also known to be big (or should we say small) ballet fans…

MENU 2

BREAKFAST

25g wholewheat cereal

1 scrambled egg on 25g toast

1 small banana

LUNCH

Pasta Salad with Fresh Vegetables (and optional goat's cheese)

2 crispbreads

2 satsumas

or

DINNER

1 portion Lamb Stew with Lentils and Spinach

large green salad

2 satsumas

MENU 3

BREAKFAST

100g strawberries (with sweetener if desired)

1 small fat-free plain yogurt

1 sandwich of 2 slices (50g) wholemeal bread and 25g low-fat hard cheese

LUNCH

Kipper and Mushroom Salad

1 wholemeal bread roll

1 large apple

or

DINNER

1 portion Pot-roasted Chicken with Cranberries

2 new potatoes

large portion lightly cooked cabbage

1 large apple

MENU 4

BREAKFAST

½ grapefruit

Porridge, sprinkled with bran and served with skimmed milk

1 bagel with low-fat spread topped with 25g smoked salmon

LUNCH

100g cold cooked chicken without skin

Marinated Mushroom and Artichoke Salad

1 pitta bread

1 banana

1 pear

or

DINNER

2-egg omelette cooked with 25g grated cheese

Tomato salad

Large green salad with 2 teaspoons French dressing

1 banana

1 pear

MENU 5

BREAKFAST

100g slice melon

1 slice (25g) wholemeal toast with 2 sardines in spring water

1 apple

LUNCH

Apricot and Rice Salad

50g low-fat cheese

2 wholemeal biscuits

1 yogurt

or

DINNER

Pork Chops with Barbecue Sauce

1 small jacket potato

Green salad

1 orange

MENU 6

BREAKFAST

100g unsweetened fruit salad

25g lean grilled bacon with 25g wholemeal toast and 2 medium grilled tomatoes

1 small fat-free yogurt

LUNCH

1 portion Mushroom and Artichoke Pizza

25g cooked rice with 25g cooked peas, ½ cooked carrot, diced, 2 chopped shallots mixed with just enough French dressing to moisten

Small bunch of grapes

2 kiwi fruit

or

DINNER

Pork tenderloin with orange sauce

50g sugar snap peas

Small bunch of grapes and 2 kiwi fruit

THE RECIPES

Three Bean Pâté

(Serves 10 – can be frozen for up to a month)

400g can flageolet beans

425g can borlotti beans

425g can cannellini beans

4–6 garlic cloves

150ml tahini paste

juice of 2 lemons

a small bunch of fresh parsley

1 teaspoon fresh thyme

salt and freshly ground black pepper

Put all the beans in a colander and rinse them thoroughly under cold running water. Peel and crush the garlic cloves. Put the garlic in a food processor with the beans, tahini paste, lemon juice, parsley and thyme, and purée.

Season the mixture with salt and pepper. Process the purée again, adding 2–3 tablespoons of hot water, until creamy. Turn into a bowl and serve or freeze.

Pasta Salad with Fresh Vegetables

(Serves 4)

350g pasta
1 red onion, peeled and sliced
1 teaspoon cider vinegar
75g small broccoli, broken into very small florets
225g small courgettes, trimmed and diced
2 sticks celery, trimmed and diced
½ cucumber, peeled and diced
2 small carrots, peeled and diced
1 large beef tomato, diced, or 8 cherry tomatoes, halved
3 tablespoons fresh basil leaves
3 tablespoons virgin olive oil
50g goat's cheese (optional)
salt and freshly ground black pepper

To pickle the onion, cover with boiling water and allow to stand for 30 seconds. Drain and return to the bowl with just enough cider vinegar to cover the slices. Store in the refrigerator to marinate for 3 hours.

Cook the pasta according to the instructions on the packet, leaving it slightly firm.

Put the broccoli florets in a pan containing just enough boiling water to cover them. Add a pinch of salt and blanch for 2 minutes. Drain and put aside.

Put the courgettes, celery, cucumber, carrots and tomatoe(s) in a serving bowl. Drain the onion and add to the bowl, along with the broccoli and basil. Mix thoroughly.

Drain and rinse the pasta in cold water, then drain again thoroughly and add to the bowl with the olive oil. Toss well and add salt and pepper to taste. Sprinkle with crumbled goat's cheese (if using) and serve cold.

Kipper and Mushroom Salad

(Serves 4)

4 large kipper fillets, skinned and cut across the grain into 5mm strips

225g mushrooms, sliced

1 small red pepper, deseeded and sliced

2 tablespoons parsley, chopped

DRESSING

juice of 1 lemon

2 teaspoons chilli sauce or ½ teaspoon Tabasco sauce

4 tablespoons single cream

3 tablespoons olive oil

freshly ground black pepper

Put the kippers in a bowl and add the mushrooms and red pepper.

Whisk the lemon juice and chilli sauce or Tabasco sauce together in another bowl. As you do so, add the cream slowly, then stir in the oil and season to taste. Pour the dressing over the kipper salad, cover and leave to marinate in the refrigerator for at least 4 hours.

When chilled, remove from the bowl using a slotted spoon and arrange in a serving dish. Whisk the remaining sauce well and pour over the salad. Garnish with chopped parsley.

Pot-roasted Chicken with Cranberries

(Serves 4)

1.4kg roasting chicken

225g cranberries

1 tablespoon raw brown sugar

rind of 1 orange, grated

juice of 2 oranges

salt and freshly ground black pepper

4 sprigs rosemary

1 tablespoon honey

Preheat the oven to 190°C/gas mark 5. You will need a covered ovenproof casserole into which the chicken will fit snugly. Put the cranberries, sugar, orange rind and juice into the casserole and mix together.

Wipe the chicken inside and out and season well, paying special attention to the inside of the chicken. Place on top of the cranberries together with the rosemary sprigs, cover and cook for one hour.

Remove the lid of the casserole and spread the honey over the chicken. Continue cooking for a further 20 minutes, basting frequently with the cooking juices until the chicken is golden-brown.

Lift the chicken from the casserole and place it on the serving dish. Discard the rosemary sprigs. Remove the cranberries with a draining spoon and arrange them around the chicken. Carefully skim off and discard any fat from the cooking juices. Serve cooking juices separately.

Apricot and Rice Salad

(Serves 4)

225g long-grain brown rice
1 red pepper, deseeded and sliced
225g dried apricots, roughly chopped
10 cm piece of cucumber, diced
75g pumpkin seeds
2 fresh apricots
parsley for garnish

DRESSING

3 tablespoons sunflower oil
1½ tablespoons sherry vinegar
1 teaspoon whole grain mustard
freshly ground black pepper

Cook the rice according to the instructions on the packet and mix the ingredients of the dressing together. Drain the rice and turn into a bowl. Add the dressing, and leave to cool for 1 hour.

Mix the peppers, apricots, cucumber and pumpkin seeds with the rice. Season to taste and garnish with the parsley.

Pork Chops with Barbecue Sauce

(Serves 4)

4 very lean pork chops
1 medium onion, roughly chopped
1 tablespoon virgin olive oil
3 teaspoons horseradish sauce
1 teaspoon mustard powder
1 teaspoon celery seeds
400g tinned tomatoes
2 tablespoons honey
1 tablespoon malt vinegar
1 tablespoon Worcestershire sauce
chopped parsley to garnish

Heat the oven to 175°C/gas mark 4. Heat the oil in a pan and sauté the onion over a medium heat for about 6 minutes until transparent. Add all the other sauce ingredients. Cover and simmer for about 10 minutes.

Trim any rind and fat from the chops and place them in an ovenproof dish large enough to hold them in a single layer. Spoon the sauce over the chops, cover and cook for 45 minutes until tender. Garnish with the parsley before serving.

Mushroom and Artichoke Pizza

(Serves 4)

225g wholewheat flour

salt and freshly ground black pepper

1 tablespoon fresh mixed herbs

1 teaspoon sugar

1 teaspoon yeast

TOPPING

225g fresh mushrooms, thinly sliced

6 spring onions, finely chopped

2 garlic cloves, finely chopped

25g butter

2 tablespoons white wine

3 tablespoons virgin olive oil

1 tablespoon fresh mixed herbs or 1 teaspoon dried herbs

salt and freshly ground black pepper

400g tin artichoke hearts in brine, drained

75g Mozzarella cheese

25g freshly grated Parmesan

Heat the oven to 220°C/gas mark 7. Grease a 200mm sandwich tin with a little olive oil. Combine the flour, ½ teaspoon of salt, a few twists of freshly ground black pepper and half the herbs in a bowl. Measure 175ml of hand-hot water into a jug, then whisk in the sugar and yeast. Leave for about 10 minutes until frothy, then stir into the dry ingredients. Mix to a smooth dough with your fingers, kneading if necessary. Press the dough into the cake tin, right up to the sides. Cover with a damp cloth and leave for 25 minutes, until risen.

Sauté the onions in 15g butter for 1 minute. Reduce the heat, add the wine and cook for 5 minutes. Remove from the pan.

Heat 1 tablespoon of the oil with the remainder of the butter and sauté the mushrooms over a fairly high heat for about 3 minutes until they are soft. Add the garlic to the mushrooms. When the mushrooms begin to release their juices, add the herbs and some seasoning. Add the onion juices and simmer until almost all the liquid has evaporated.

Push the dough lightly back up to the side of the tin if it has slipped, then spread the onions on the pizza. Grate the Mozzarella and sprinkle over the onions. Spread the mushrooms over the cheese and lay the artichoke pieces in a pattern among the mushrooms. Sprinkle with the Parmesan. Dribble the remaining olive oil over the pizza and sprinkle on the remaining fresh herbs. Bake in the oven for 20 minutes and serve at once.

Pork Tenderloin with Orange Sauce

(Serves 4)

450g very lean pork tenderloin
5 teaspoons vegetable oil
3 sheets filo pastry
parsley to garnish

STUFFING

50g dried peaches, chopped
50g bacon, finely chopped
1 small onion, finely chopped
1 tablespoon vegetable oil
1 tablespoon freshly chopped parsley
15g pistachio nuts, finely chopped
50g fresh breadcrumbs

SAUCE

1 orange
450ml chicken stock
2 teaspoons arrowroot powder
2 spring onions
1 tablespoon Grand Marnier or Cointreau (optional)
1 teaspoon lemon juice
salt and freshly ground black pepper

Heat the oven to 200°C/gas mark 6. Trim any fat and sinew from the meat. Make a deep cut along the length of the meat and open it out. Place the meat on a sheet of plastic film and lay another sheet over it. Using the end of a rolling pin or a wooden mallet, beat the meat from the centre out to the sides until it is quite thin, then set aside.

Cover the peaches with boiling water. Heat the oil in a small pan and sauté the onion over a moderate heat for 4 minutes, then add the bacon and cook for a further 4 minutes. Add the parsley, pistachio nuts, peaches and breadcrumbs. Season with salt and pepper.

Uncover the pork and lay the stuffing along its length. Fold the ends in and then the sides and tie securely, at intervals, with string.

Heat 3 teaspoons of the oil in a frying pan and cook the pork over a high heat to seal in the juices, turning the pork to make sure that all sides are sealed. Leave to cool at room temperature for about 1 hour, then carefully remove the string.

Lay the sheets of filo pastry on top of each other and place the pork on top, in the centre. Fold over the ends and then roll the pork in the pastry. Place on a lightly oiled baking tray. Brush with the remaining oil and sprinkle with water. Bake for 30 minutes until crisp and golden.

In the meantime, pare the rind of the orange thinly, cut into fine matchstick strips and set aside. Cut the orange in half, squeeze the juice and pour it into a small pan with the stock. Bring to the boil and continue to boil uncovered until the juice has been reduced to 285ml.

Mix the arrowroot with 1 tablespoon of water until smooth, and stir into the orange mixture. Simmer until thickened. Slice the spring onions very finely and add them to the sauce with the optional liqueur, the lemon juice and the orange strips. Simmer for 2 minutes, then season to taste. Pour into a warmed sauceboat.

Slice the pork with a very sharp knife, serve with the sauce and garnish with the parsley.

Marinated Mushroom and Artichoke Salad

(Serves 4)

450g small white button mushrooms
225g can artichoke hearts
3 tablespoons lemon juice
2 teaspoons coriander seeds
½ teaspoon cumin seeds
1 garlic clove, peeled
2 tablespoons virgin olive oil
2 tablespoons cider vinegar
2 tablespoons clear honey
2 tablespoons fresh coriander, chopped
red onion, sliced into rings
white onion, sliced into rings
salt and freshly ground black pepper
fresh coriander for garnish

Trim the base of the mushroom stalks and wipe them clean. Drain the artichoke hearts and put them in a large bowl.

Bring a saucepan of water to the boil, add 1 tablespoon of lemon juice and the mushrooms. Cook in boiling water for 1 minute. Drain the mushrooms and rinse them in cold water. Drain again, pat dry and add them to the artichokes.

Crush the coriander seeds, cumin seeds and the garlic, using a mortar and pestle. Heat 1 tablespoon of the oil in a pan, add the crushed mixture and stir-fry gently for 1 minute. Add the remaining lemon juice, the vinegar and honey, and stir-fry for a further 2 minutes. Pour the mixture over the mushrooms and artichokes, add the remaining oil and stir until the mushrooms are coated. Add the chopped coriander, and salt and pepper to taste, and stir again. Cover and chill in the refrigerator for 4 hours, stirring occasionally.

Arrange the onion rings around the edge of a serving dish. Toss the mushrooms and artichokes well and spoon them into the centre. The salad can be left covered to marinate for up to 24 hours.

Beef and Pork Goulash

(Serves 4)

250g rump steak, cut into cubes
250g lean pork, cut into cubes
2 medium onions, roughly chopped
1 red pepper, deseeded and chopped
2 tablespoon virgin olive oil
2 level teaspoons paprika
3 tablespoons tomato paste
250ml stock
2 large tomatoes, skinned and quartered
a bouquet garni
150ml beer
2 teaspoons ground arrowroot slaked in 2 tablespoons water
salt and freshly ground black pepper

Heat the oven to 160°C/gas mark 3. Fry the onions and pepper lightly in the oil for 3–4 minutes. Add the meat and fry lightly on all sides for about 5 minutes, until golden brown. Add the paprika and fry for about 1 minute longer. Stir in the tomato paste, salt and pepper and cook for a further minute.

Add the stock, tomatoes and bouquet garni. Put the mixture in a casserole and cook for about an hour until the meat is tender. Add the beer and cook for a few minutes longer. Remove the bouquet garni and stir the arrowroot into the dish to thicken.

Lamb Stew with Lentils and Spinach

(Serves 4)

450g shoulder of lamb, trimmed and cut into 25mm cubes
225g green or brown lentils, washed in cold water
450g fresh spinach, well washed
1 onion, finely sliced
2 garlic cloves, finely sliced
2 carrots, sliced
40g butter
1 tablespoon virgin olive oil
400g can peeled tomatoes
2 dried chilli peppers (optional)
½ teaspoon cumin
½ teaspoon ground coriander
2 tablespoons parsley or coriander, freshly chopped
salt and freshly ground black pepper

Place 15g of the butter and the olive oil in a large flameproof casserole. Heat until the butter melts and sizzles, then add the lamb cubes, stirring until they are sealed and brown. Leaving the fat in the casserole, remove the lamb with a slotted spoon and put aside.

Add the onion, garlic and carrots to the casserole and cook over a moderate heat until soft. Add the tomatoes, lamb cubes, 1 teaspoon of salt, ½ teaspoon pepper, chillies (if using), lentils and enough water to just cover the mixture. Stir in the cumin and simmer for 1¼ hours, until the lentils are cooked. Add a little more water if the mixture begins to dry. When cooked, set the mixture aside.

Cook the spinach in the remaining 25g of butter with a little salt and the ground coriander. Reheat the lentil mixture and stir in the cooked spinach. Garnish with the chopped parsley or coriander and serve.

FAMOUS PEOPLE DON'T GET FAT

Sarah Jessica Parker keeps her size-six figure in shape by walking, cycling and rollerblading around New York. Simple as that!

Davina McCall

SEXY DAVINA McCall never seems to leave our TV screens during the long summer months – good for her that she often seems to look substantially more fabulous than some of the *Big Brother* housemates! Davina recently gave birth to her second child, but unlike some celebrities we could name, she did not resort to crash dieting in order to regain her figure. Nevertheless, she now weighs less than she did before she started her pregnancy, and that makes her feel more self-confident than ever before.

The secret of Davina's slimness is down to good, old-fashioned hard work. She concentrates on eating healthily and avoiding the junk, and follows a few very simple rules:

- Don't skip meals. If you do, you'll be more likely to snack.

- Avoid carbs after lunch.

- When you do eat carbs, only eat 'good' carbs – so up your intake of wholewheat pasta and rice, and no more white bread.

- Eat plenty of protein.

- Eat five portions of fruit and vegetables every day.

In the pages that follow are some recipes that will help you get a figure like Davina's. They are generally high in protein and low in carbs, and the carbs included are 'good' carbs; you will find that there are a wide range of fruit and vegetables used in the recipes, making it easier for you to fulfil your five-a-day quota; and some of the recipes are rather special, meaning that you can bring a bit of Davina's celebrity glamour into your own life!

Crudités with Tofu Mayonnaise

(Serves 6)

175g celeriac
4 tablespoons virgin olive oil
juice and grated zest of ½ lemon
175g small courgettes
juice and grated zest of ½ lime
1 tablespoon cardamom seeds
175g carrots
juice and grated zest of ½ orange
175g raw or cooked beetroot
2 teaspoons cider vinegar
1 tablespoon finely chopped fresh dill or 1 teaspoon dried
salt
freshly ground white pepper
freshly ground black pepper

DRESSING

300g firm tofu
2 tablespoons virgin olive oil
2 tablespoons lemon juice
2 garlic cloves
salt and freshly ground black pepper

Make the tofu mayonnaise by processing all the ingredients until smooth. Add salt and pepper to taste then turn into a serving bowl. Cover and chill.

Peel and grate the celeriac, then toss in a dressing made with 1 tablespoon olive oil, the grated lemon rind and juice and salt and white pepper to taste. Top and tail the courgettes and cut them into sticks. Place in a bowl and toss in a dressing made of 1 tablespoon of the olive oil, the grated lime rind and juice and seasoning.

Dry fry the cardamom seeds in a non-stick pan for about 2 minutes until toasted, then crush in a mortar and pestle, removing the husks. Peel and grate the carrots and place in a bowl, mixing them with a dressing made from 1 tablespoon of olive oil, the orange juice and zest and the crushed cardamom seeds, adding salt and freshly ground black pepper to taste.

Peel and grate the beetroot and toss in a dressing made of 1 tablespoon olive oil, the cider vinegar, dill and salt and freshly ground white pepper to taste.

Arrange neat mounds of all 4 vegetables separately on individual plates, draining them with a slotted spoon if too wet. Serve the tofu mayonnaise separately as a dip.

Warm Duck Salad

(Serves 6)

2 duck breasts

2 tablespoons virgin olive oil

15g unsalted butter

12 medium mushrooms, wiped and thinly sliced

1 garlic clove, peeled and sliced

½ teaspoon balsamic or cider vinegar

1 tablespoon lemon juice

1 small radicchio lettuce

1 bunch watercress

1 head of curly endive or escarole

1 tablespoon chopped parsley

1 tablespoon chopped basil

MARINADE

2 shallots or 1 small onion, finely chopped

1 tablespoon lemon juice

1 tablespoon virgin olive oil

1 tablespoon fresh mixed herbs

salt and freshly ground black pepper

Skin the duck breasts and cut them into long, thin strips. Mix all the marinade ingredients in a bowl and season well. Place the duck strips in the marinade, cover and chill for at least 1 hour.

Drain the duck. Heat the oil and butter in a pan, add the duck and sauté for 2–3 minutes. Quickly transfer the duck to a separate dish and add the mushrooms to the pan, with a little more butter if necessary. Sauté for 2–3 minutes over a high heat, stirring occasionally. Add the marinade to the mushrooms with the garlic, vinegar and lemon juice. Reduce the mixture in the pan by boiling for 2 minutes. Return the duck to the pan, coating each strip with the mixture, then remove from the heat.

Wash and dry the mixed salad leaves, divide them between plates and top with the duck strips. Pour the dressing over the salads and garnish with the parsley and basil. Serve at once.

Carrot, Tomato and Cardamom Soup

(Serves 4)

1½ tablespoons sunflower oil

1 onion, finely chopped

275g carrots, peeled and roughly chopped

275g fresh tomatoes, skinned, seeded and roughly chopped

975ml vegetable or chicken stock

9 cardamom pods, crushed and tied in a piece of muslin (pods and seeds)

salt and freshly ground black pepper

chopped coriander or parsley for garnish

Heat the oil in a large saucepan and cook the onion over a medium heat until transparent. Add the carrots and tomatoes and stir for 2–3 minutes. Add the stock and cardamom pods and bring to the boil. Reduce the heat and simmer for about 30 minutes until the carrots are tender. Remove the cardamom from the saucepan and leave to cool, then squeeze the muslin over the pan to extract all the juices.

Purée the soup in a food processor or blender, then return to the saucepan and reheat gently. Season and garnish with the chopped herbs.

Marinated Cod

(Serves 4)

1 bay leaf

2 tablespoons virgin olive oil

juice of 1 lemon

1–2 garlic cloves

2 teaspoons ground coriander

salt and freshly ground black pepper

900g cod fillet

4 lime wedges and fresh parsley to garnish

To make the marinade, tear the bay leaf into three pieces. Place the bay leaf, oil, lemon juice, peeled garlic, coriander and seasoning in a shallow dish and whisk together with a fork. Cut the fish into four pieces and immerse, skin side up, in the marinade. Leave to marinate for at least 2 hours, turning and basting two or three times.

Preheat the grill. Place the pieces of fish in an ovenproof dish, skin side down, and spoon over the remaining marinade. Cook for 10 minutes under a moderately hot grill, basting occasionally with the marinade until the fish is golden brown. Arrange on a serving dish, garnish with the lime wedges and parsley and serve with a green salad.

Banana and Raspberry Smoothie

(Serves 4)
120g bananas
180g frozen raspberries
mint to garnish

Blend together the banana and the unthawed raspberries in a food processor until you have a smooth purée. Pour into 4 small glasses and garnish with the mint.

Mussels in White Wine

(Serves 4)
1.8kg bag of mussels
2 garlic cloves
2 sticks celery
2 shallots
2 tablespoons virgin olive oil
150ml dry white wine
2 tablespoons chopped fresh parsley
2 tablespoons chopped celery leaves
freshly ground black pepper

Discard any mussels that have open shells. Scrub and wash the remainder to remove any barnacles, grit or weed. Gently pull out the hairy beard on each mussel and discard. Place the mussels in a large saucepan. Add at least 285ml water, cover tightly and cook over a high heat for 3–5 minutes, shaking from time to time, until the shells open. You may need to cook the mussels in batches.

When all the shells are open, remove them from the pan, discarding any with closed shells. Strain the cooking liquid through fine muslin and reserve.

Finely chop the garlic, celery and shallots. Heat the oil in a saucepan and sauté the chopped vegetables for 5 minutes. Add the liquid from the mussels and the white wine and bring to the boil. Add the mussels, cover and simmer for 3–4 minutes.

Serve the mussels and sauce in soup plates. Sprinkle with freshly chopped herbs and a generous helping of black pepper.

Quick Spaghetti Carbonara

(Serves 4)

450g wholewheat spaghetti

1 medium onion

1 tablespoon virgin olive oil

8 rashers smoked bacon

115g mature cheddar or fresh parmesan cheese

3 eggs

3 tablespoons milk

3 tablespoons fresh parsley, chopped

salt and freshly ground black pepper

Cook the pasta according to the packet instructions until al dente. Meanwhile, peel and chop the onion. Heat the oil in a pan and briefly fry the bacon until just cooked on both sides. Remove, leaving the cooking juices behind. Add the onion and cook for 4 minutes over a medium heat until softened and beginning to turn golden. Cut the bacon into large squares. Grate the cheese on to a plate, then beat the eggs thoroughly in a small bowl.

Drain the cooked spaghetti and return to the pan. Quickly stir in the beaten eggs, the grated cheese and the onion and bacon mixture. Stir in the parsley and season well. Serve immediately on warmed plates.

Lebanese Cucumber Soup

(Serves 4)

1 medium cucumber

2 spring onions

1 garlic clove

225ml carton natural low-fat yoghurt

75ml sour cream

1 tablespoon chopped fresh mint

mint sprigs for garnish

1 pinch ground cumin

1 teaspoon lemon juice

salt and freshly ground black pepper

Reserving a small amount of cucumber to garnish, peel the rest and finely grate or chop it over a bowl to catch any liquid. Trim the spring onions and finely chop the bulbs and about 80mm of the green stalk. Crush and finely chop the garlic.

Mix the grated or chopped cucumber and its liquid with all the other ingredients and stir well until smooth. Season to taste with salt and black pepper. Chill the soup mixture until required, then divide into 4 bowls, garnish with sprigs of fresh mint and thin slices of cucumber.

Pan-fried Steak with Green Peppercorn Sauce

(Serves 4)

4 x 175g sirloin steaks

2 shallots

1 teaspoon green peppercorns, crushed

2 teaspoons coarse grain mustard

2 tablespoons brandy

225ml strained Greek yoghurt or 150ml single cream

juice of ½ lemon

salt and freshly ground black pepper

Trim any excess fat from the steaks. Place some of the fat into a non-stick frying pan and cook over a medium heat to render it. Discard any solid fat. Raise the heat to high and fry the steaks in the pan for 2 minutes each side. Reduce the heat and cook for up to 2–3 more minutes each side. Eight minutes will give a well-done steak; reduce the cooking time by half for rare meat. Remove the steaks and keep warm.

Chop the shallots finely and add to the pan juices. Cook over a low heat, stirring until lightly coloured. Add the crushed peppercorns, mustard and brandy. Stir in the yoghurt or cream and lemon juice, then heat gently before serving with the steaks.

Figs with Prosciutto and Goat's Cheese

(Serves 4)

4 fresh, ripe figs

4 slices prosciutto

115g soft goat's cheese

50g fromage frais

12 fresh basil leaves

Carefully slice the figs into fan shapes with a sharp, serrated knife, and arrange on the plates with the slices of ham. Combine the goat's cheese and fromage frais by mashing with a fork until smooth. Tear 4 basil leaves into small strips and stir into the cheese. Divide the mixture into round portions and arrange them on the plates. Garnish with the remaining basil leaves and serve immediately.

Mexican Trout

(Serves 4)

2 tablespoons olive oil

1 large onion, thinly sliced

1 dessertspoon white wine vinegar

1 red pepper, seeded and diced

juice of 2 limes

3 tablespoons chopped parsley

2 dashes Tabasco sauce

4 small trout, gutted

salt and freshly ground black pepper

AVOCADO DIP

1 ripe avocado

1 tablespoon natural yoghurt

Preheat the oven to 180°C/gas mark 4.

Heat the oil in a frying pan, add the onion and vinegar and cook over a moderate heat for 5 minutes. Add the pepper and cook for a further 2 minutes. Add the juice of one of the limes, 2 tablespoons of the parsley and the Tabasco. Mix thoroughly and remove from the heat.

Brush an ovenproof dish with a little oil, place the trout in the dish and season lightly. Spoon over the onion and pepper mixture. Tightly cover the dish with foil and bake in the oven for about 20 minutes.

Halve the avocado, remove the stone and peel away the skin. Blend the flesh with the juice of the second lime and the yoghurt. Garnish the baked trout and the dip with the remaining parsley. Serve the dip with the fish or in a separate dish.

Asparagus with Orange Dressing

(Serves 4)

450g fresh asparagus

grated peel of orange

3 tablespoons orange juice

1 tablespoon lemon juice

¼ teaspoon mustard powder

3 tablespoons virgin olive oil

1 spring onion

1 small bunch parsley

salt and freshly ground black pepper

1 orange for garnish

Prepare the asparagus by rinsing and removing the base of any tough stems.

Blanch the asparagus in boiling salted water and immediately plunge into iced water to retain the colour. Keep on one side. Bring 150ml water to the boil in a small pan. Add the grated orange peel and boil for 3 minutes. Remove the peel and mix it with the orange and lemon juice, salt, pepper, mustard powder and oil. Finely chop the spring onion and 1 tablespoon of parsley. Mix well.

Peel the orange, cutting away all the pith, and slice out individual segments by cutting against each side of the segment's skin. Plunge the blanched asparagus into boiling water until just cooked. Drain well.

Put the asparagus on individual plates and pour the dressing over evenly. Garnish with sprigs of parsley, orange segments and very thin strips of orange peel, if desired.

Wilted Spinach Omelette

(Serves 4)

450g fresh spinach
25g butter
1 small onion
1 garlic clove
1 tablespoon olive oil
8 eggs
2 teaspoons grated nutmeg
¼ teaspoon salt
freshly ground black pepper
2 tablespoons chopped parsley

Wash the spinach and put it into a large pan with 4 tablespoons of water and the butter. Cook over a medium-high heat for 2–3 minutes, stirring continually until the spinach has just wilted. Then leave it to drain in a colander.

Chop the onion and crush the garlic clove. Heat the oil in a large pan over a moderate heat and add the onion and garlic. Cook for 7 minutes until softened and golden.

In the meantime, roughly chop the spinach and squeeze out any excess water. Beat the eggs well with 5 tablespoons of water, the nutmeg and the seasoning. Add the spinach to the onions and spread evenly over the pan. Pour the eggs over the vegetables and cook for 2–3 minutes. Carefully lift up the edges of the omelette with a spatula to allow any uncooked egg to run underneath. As soon as the omelette is firm and its underside is golden, fold it over in half with the spatula and turn on to a plate. Divide into four portions and garnish with the parsley.

Stuffed Mushrooms

(Serves 4)

275g large open-cup mushrooms or flat field mushrooms

2 garlic cloves

finely grated rind of 1 lemon

40g wholemeal breadcrumbs

1 tablespoon fresh chopped marjoram

1 tablespoon fresh chopped parsley

3 tablespoons virgin olive oil

salt and freshly ground black pepper

parsley sprigs and lemon wedges for garnish

Preheat the oven to 180°C/gas mark 4.

Wipe the mushrooms with a damp cloth. Remove the stalks and chop them finely. Crush the garlic and place in a bowl together with the lemon rind, the chopped stalks, breadcrumbs, herbs and 1½ tablespoons of the olive oil. Add salt and the pepper to taste, then stir well to mix all the ingredients.

Brush the bottom of a shallow ovenproof dish with 2 teaspoons of oil. Arrange the mushrooms and sprinkle over the remaining oil. Bake in the oven for 15 minutes. Serve hot, garnished with fresh herbs and lemon wedges.

Chicken Simmered with Spicy Dried Fruit

(Serves 4)

4 x 275g chicken pieces

285ml chicken stock

150ml orange juice

2 teaspoons paprika

2 teaspoons ground ginger

½ teaspoon ground cinnamon

¼ teaspoon ground allspice

250g packet ready-to-eat dried fruit salad

salt and freshly ground black pepper

Remove the skin and any fat from the chicken. Pour the stock and the orange juice into a flameproof casserole, then add the spices and stir it well. Add the dried fruit and bring slowly to the boil, stirring continuously. Add the chicken and season to taste. Baste the pieces of chicken well with the liquid.

Lower the heat, cover the pan with a tight-fitting lid and simmer very gently for about 30–35 minutes until the chicken is tender. Lift the lid occasionally during the cooking and stir the chicken and fruit to ensure that they cook evenly. Season the dish to taste and serve immediately.

Prawn and Mango Cocktail

(Serves 4)

1 large ripe mango

1 lime

½ sweet red pepper

½ sweet yellow pepper

1 teaspoon finely chopped green or red chilli

2 tablespoons chopped coriander or parsley

225g peeled prawns

2 tablespoons virgin olive oil

1 little gem lettuce

Peel the mango, remove the stone and chop finely. Juice the lime and core and dice the peppers.

Put the mango, lime juice, peppers, chopped chilli and herbs in a bowl, then add the prawns and marinate in the fridge for 2 hours. Drain the liquid and mix it with the olive oil to make a dressing. Wash, dry and shred the lettuce, adding some dressing. Divide between four bowls and pile the prawns, mango and peppers on the top.

Mangetout and Bacon Salad

(Serves 4)

2 slices wholemeal bread, crusts removed and cut into cubes

6–8 rashers lean back bacon, rind and any excess fat removed

450g mangetout

DRESSING

1½ tablespoons virgin olive oil or hazelnut oil

½ tablespoon white wine vinegar

salt and freshly ground black pepper

Pre-heat the oven to 190°C/gas mark 5.

Spread the bread cubes on a baking sheet and brown lightly in the oven for about 12 minutes. Cut the bacon into 15mm wide strips. Cook in a dry non-stick frying pan over a moderate heat until crisp and lightly golden. Keep warm.

Whisk the dressing ingredients in a small bowl and bring a saucepan of water to the boil. Add the mangetout to the boiling water and cook for 3–4 minutes until the pods are tender but still crunchy. Plunge the mangetout into ice-cold water to keep them crisp, then pat dry.

Pour the dressing into a warmed serving bowl, add the mangetout, bacon and croutons, season to taste and toss well together. This salad is particularly delicious served warm.

Haddock Fillets with Coriander and Orange

(Serves 4)

4 x 175g pieces skinned haddock fillet

1 tablespoon plain flour

1 tablespoon sesame seeds

2 tablespoons ground coriander seeds

finely grated rind and juice of 1 large orange

15g unsalted butter

1 tablespoon virgin olive oil

salt and freshly ground black pepper

285ml fish stock

1 teaspoon cornflour

4 tablespoons single cream

Pre-heat the oven to 200°C/gas mark 6.

Wash and pat dry the fish portions and season them. Mix the flour, sesame seeds, coriander and orange rind together and coat the fish with the mixture.

Heat the butter and oil together and brush half the mixture lightly on to a non-stick baking tray. Arrange the fish on the tray and pour the remaining butter and oil over the top. Bake in the oven for 15 minutes.

Pour the stock and orange juice into a wide shallow pan. Boil the mixture to reduce by half. Mix the cornflour and 2 tablespoons of water into a smooth paste, stir in the cream, then slowly add to the stock, stirring until thickened. Arrange the fish on a serving plate and serve the sauce separately.

Broccoli, Almond and Nutmeg Soup

(Serves 6)

450g broccoli, trimmed and divided into florets
1 medium onion, chopped
1 medium potato, peeled and diced
2 ½ tablespoons virgin olive oil
850ml vegetable or chicken stock
75g flaked almonds
285ml semi-skimmed milk
1 generous pinch nutmeg
salt and freshly ground black pepper

Reserve 50g of the broccoli florets and roughly chop the remainder. Heat 2 tablespoons of oil in a saucepan and cook the onion over a medium heat until transparent. Add the potato and chopped broccoli along with the stock. Bring to the boil and simmer for 20 minutes until the potatoes are tender. Remove from the heat.

Heat the rest of the oil in a frying pan and add the flaked almonds, stirring gently. Remove as soon as they are golden brown. Reserve some almonds for garnish and put the rest in a blender with the vegetables and their liquid. Blend until smooth. Return to the saucepan, add the milk and reheat. Add the nutmeg and season.

Break the remaining broccoli into small florets, cook in 150ml of boiling water for 2–3 minutes and drain the water into the soup. Garnish each bowl of soup with the florets and the reserved almonds.

Demi Moore

WHEN SEXY Demi Moore had to get in trim for her raunchy role in the film *Striptease*, she took advice from real-life strippers and topless dancers. Not all of us can do that – or would necessarily want to – but there are other slimming secrets we can learn from Demi.

She follows a regime of eating raw food, which is a good dieting plan in all sorts of ways. Firstly, it means that your food intake will naturally be inclined towards fruit and vegetables, which, as we all know, are not only great for slimmers but also the healthiest option. The other theory of the raw-food diet is that if you cook food at above 118°C, the heat destroys certain enzymes which aid digestion. If you eat the food raw, your body can process it more quickly and so you put on less weight.

The details of the raw-food diet are:

- 75 per cent of the food you consume must be raw.
- The remaining food you consume must be cooked at a temperature of under 118°C.
- Everything that you eat should be vegetarian and, where possible, organic.

There is no reason why this diet should be anything less than delicious, and it should enable you to lose 1–2kg a week. Below are a few suggestions of recipes you could try on this diet – and remember to use organic ingredients wherever possible.

RECIPE 1

Mix together 50g grated carrot, 50g shredded cabbage, 1 chopped apple, 25g chopped walnuts and 1 tablespoon of mayonnaise to make a delicious coleslaw with a twist.

RECIPE 2

Top 50g lightly cooked pasta with some freshly puréed tomatoes. Sprinkle with 25g vegetarian cheese for an authentic Italian treat.

RECIPE 3

Make an enormous salad from loads of green leaves and plenty of healthy watercress, a large, juicy tomato, cucumber, celery, 25g almonds, some satsuma segments and a small chopped apple. Dress with salt, pepper and freshly squeezed orange juice.

RECIPE 4

Braise 100g celery in gently simmering water and cover with a cheese sauce made from organic skimmed milk and organic low-fat cheese. Serve with raw broccoli and cauliflower florets.

RECIPE 5

Top a huge, healthy portion of wilted spinach with 2 lightly poached fresh eggs. Serve with a side salad of grated carrot and orange segments.

RECIPE 6

For a salad with a difference, combine 25g bean sprouts, 25g alfalfa sprouts, ¼ chopped red pepper and 25g chopped radish. Dress with lemon juice, a little crushed garlic and ½ teaspoon tahini mixed with ½ teaspoon olive oil. Serve with chopped parsley and lemon wedges, and perhaps add a side salad of sliced red onions and sliced cucumber.

Gwyneth Paltrow

IN THE hit film *Shallow Hal*, Gwyneth Paltrow went the opposite way to most Hollywood stars and had to make herself look overweight!

Of course, the reality is very different, and Gwyneth has a figure that most of us dream of. She follows a very strict macrobiotic diet, the health benefits of which are very well documented. The rules are:

- 60 per cent of your food intake must comprise whole grains such as brown rice and pulses.

- The rest of your diet comprises vegetables (except potatoes) and fish.

- You are not allowed to consume meat, dairy products, processed food, alcohol or caffeine.

This is originally an oriental diet, and it works on a number of levels: on the lowest level you can eat any of the allowed foods, while on the highest level you can only eat brown rice and water. For a sensible, maintained weight-loss programme you should really just follow the lowest level, and here are a few recipes to get you on your way. *Be aware that this diet is very low in calcium and some other vitamins, so if you are going to follow it for any length of time, a calcium and vitamin supplement is important. Your local health food shop should be able to advise you on this.*

Fruit and Nut Risotto

(Serves 4)

350g easy-cook brown rice

250g packet ready-to-eat mixed dried fruit, roughly chopped

3 celery sticks, roughly chopped

1 large onion, finely chopped

2½ tablespoons groundnut oil or sunflower oil

½ teaspoon ground cinnamon

½ teaspoon ground ginger

1–2 tablespoons fresh coriander, chopped

90g mixture of sunflower seeds and nuts

salt and freshly ground black pepper

Heat the oil in a large pan. Add the onion and celery and cook over a gentle heat, stirring frequently for about 8 minutes, until the vegetables are soft and golden, but not brown. Add the chopped fruit and 850ml of water. Bring to the boil, cover the pan and simmer for 10 minutes.

Add the rice, salt, pepper, cinnamon and ginger, and stir to mix thoroughly. Cover and cook over a low to moderate heat until the rice is cooked and all the liquid has been absorbed.

Fold in the sunflower seeds and nuts and half the coriander. Adjust the seasoning. Transfer to a serving bowl, sprinkle with the remaining coriander and serve immediately.

Spaghetti con Cozze

(Serves 4)

1.1kg mussels
150ml fish stock
4 shallots, finely chopped
1 garlic clove, crushed
1 stick celery, chopped
1 teaspoon caster sugar
4 tablespoons parsley, chopped
1 tablespoon olive oil
400g wholemeal spaghetti
salt and freshly ground black pepper

Wash the mussels thoroughly in two or three changes of cold water. Remove the beards and discard any shells that are broken. Sharply tap the mussels one by one and throw them away if they do not close. Leave the remaining mussels to soak in cold water for 2–4 hours to remove any sand or grit.

Pour the fish stock into a large pan. Add the shallots, garlic, celery, sugar and half the chopped parsley. Simmer gently for 5 minutes. Increase the heat, add the mussels, cover the pan and cook for a further 5 minutes, shaking the pan continuously until all the shells are open. Remove and discard any shells that remain closed.

Bring a large pan of unsalted water to the boil. Add the olive oil and spaghetti and cook until al dente.

Meanwhile, tip the cooked mussels into a muslin-lined colander, reserving the juice. Boil the juice for a few minutes until it has been reduced by half. Remove the mussels from their shells, setting aside a few unshelled ones to garnish.

Drain the spaghetti and tip it back into the pan, together with the reduced mussel juice, and cook gently for 2 minutes. Add the mussels and the other half of the parsley, mix well and add salt and pepper to taste. Divide between warmed soup bowls, garnish with the reserved mussels and serve.

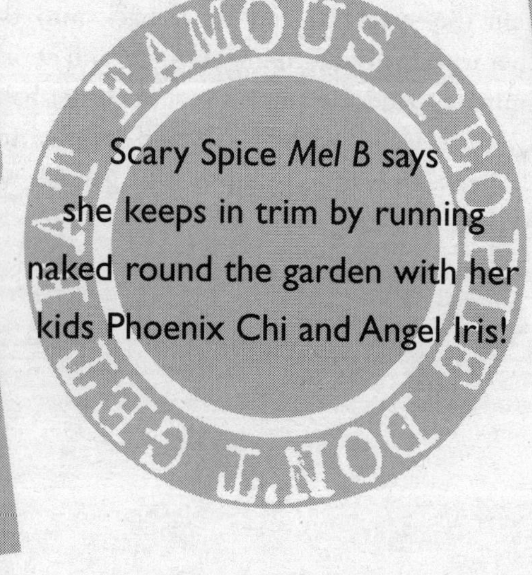

Scary Spice *Mel B* says she keeps in trim by running naked round the garden with her kids Phoenix Chi and Angel Iris!

Baby Spice *Emma Bunton* is a blue belt in karate and keeps in trim with all the exercise that practising her martial art entails. So if you really really want a celebrity figure, just follow Emma's lead.

Tomato, Orange and Fennel Salad with Trout Fillets

(Serves 4)

6 medium-ripe tomatoes, skinned, cored and sliced into thin rings
4 small oranges, peeled and with pith removed, and sliced into rings
1 bulb fennel, sliced into very thin rings
2 tablespoons orange juice
2 tablespoons lemon juice
2 tablespoons virgin olive oil
2 tablespoons fresh basil
½ teaspoon French mustard
½ teaspoon caster sugar
basil leaves for garnish
8 small trout fillets
1 lemon
2 tablespoons cucumber, chopped
salt and freshly ground black pepper

When preparing the oranges, catch any juice in a bowl and reserve it for the dressing. When preparing the fennel, reserve the fronds to garnish. Arrange the tomato, orange and fennel alternately on individual plates.

Add the measured orange juice to that collected in

the bowl, together with the lemon juice, olive oil, basil, mustard and sugar. Add salt and pepper to taste and beat well with a fork. Drizzle the mixture over the salad and allow it to stand in a cool place for 30 minutes so that the salad absorbs the flavours of the dressing. Just before serving the salad, garnish with the fennel fronds and basil leaves.

Season the fish and sprinkle with the juice of the lemon. Lightly steam the fish and, when cooked, garnish with the chopped cucumber. Serve with the salad and seeded bread (available from health stores and some supermarkets).

Spicy Lentil Soup

(Serves 4)

115g red lentils
50g carrots, finely diced
115g red kidney beans (canned)
1 small onion, finely chopped
1 tablespoon virgin olive oil
1 teaspoon cumin powder
2 teaspoons coriander powder
1 teaspoon turmeric
1 dried red chilli
1.1 litres vegetable stock
salt and freshly ground black pepper
parsley or coriander leaves for garnish

Wash the lentils thoroughly in cold water, drain and put aside. Heat the oil in a large saucepan, add the onions and cook until soft. Add the spices and cook for 2–3 minutes, stirring continuously.

Put the carrots in the saucepan with the lentils and stock. Bring to the boil, reduce the heat and simmer for 1 hour until tender. Put the rinsed kidney beans into the pan for the last 15 minutes. Garnish with parsley or coriander. Serve with wholegrain bread.

Bean Salad with Tuna

(Serves 4)

200g canned tuna in spring water
2 x 400g canned flageolet beans
1 small red onion, thinly sliced
2 tablespoons parsley, freshly chopped
radicchio or lettuce leaves for garnish

DRESSING

1 lemon
2 tablespoons virgin olive oil
salt and freshly ground black pepper

Rinse the beans thoroughly and drain. Place them in a large serving bowl and put aside. Combine the ingredients for the dressing and pour over the beans, tossing well. Drain the tuna and flake it, then fold it gently into the beans, together with the onion. Add the chopped parsley and salt and pepper to taste. Spoon on the tuna and beans, garnish with the radicchio or lettuce, and serve.

Salmon with Brown Rice

(Serves 4)

350g fresh salmon fillets
350g brown rice
1 green pepper, finely diced
3 celery sticks, finely chopped
1 small onion, finely chopped
2 tablespoons groundnut oil
850ml fish stock
juice of 1 small lemon
2 teaspoons curry powder
¼ teaspoon cayenne pepper
2 tablespoons parsley, freshly chopped
salt and freshly ground black pepper
2 hard boiled eggs

Rinse the rice and put aside to drain. Heat the oil in a large pan. Add the chopped vegetables and cook over a moderate heat for 10–15 minutes, stirring frequently, until soft. Meanwhile, heat the stock in a separate pan.

Add the curry powder and cayenne pepper to the vegetables and stir constantly for 2 minutes. Stir in the rice, then slowly stir in the hot stock. Bring to the boil, stirring constantly, reduce the heat and add salt and black pepper to taste. Cover and simmer until the rice is tender but still firm to the bite and almost all the stock has been absorbed.

Put the fish in a frying pan, skin side down and in a single layer. Pour the lemon juice and add enough water to just cover the fish. Season with pepper to taste and bring to a simmer. Cover and cook gently for about 8 minutes, basting occasionally, until cooked. Remove the fish from the liquid and flake into large pieces over a plate, discarding the skin and bones.

When the rice is cooked, remove the pan from the heat and gently fold in the flaked fish and the parsley. Adjust the seasoning and transfer to a serving dish. Garnish with the eggs cut into quarters. Serve immediately.

FAMOUS PEOPLE DON'T GET FAT

WAG *Charlotte Mears* keeps up with footballing fiancé Jermain Defoe with some sparring in the boxing ring and floor exercises to keep toned.

Dolly Parton

WHILE CERTAIN areas of Dolly Parton are larger than average, these days her stomach isn't one of them. And yet she still manages to eat all her favourite foods. How? By using the dieter's greatest weapon – portion control. Put simply, if you eat less food, you'll put on less weight.

Of course, portion control isn't always easy. But here are a handful of tips you can follow to help you on your way:

- A smaller plate makes less food look like more.

- If you drink a couple of large glasses of water before you eat, not only will it be very good for you, it will also help suppress your appetite.

- Try to stick rigidly to three meals per day – no snacking!

- Don't think that missing breakfast is necessarily a good idea. If you eat a sensible breakfast soon after you wake up, it will mean you are less inclined to snack mid-morning.

- If you must snack, eat fruit which is low in calories and healthy. Try celery sticks, cucumber sticks, tangerines or an apple.

Julia Roberts

AS ONE of the most gorgeous stars Hollywood has ever produced, pretty woman Julia Roberts surely has a thing or two to tell us mere mortals about slimming! Of course, she has her own slimming secrets – drinking eight glasses of water every day is a good idea of hers that we should all follow whether we're slimming or not. And she tries to eat organically wherever possible (see the appendix for more on this). But Julia, like all of us, has her own weaknesses – in her case, breakfast!

But a love of the big breakfast needn't necessarily be an obstacle to the slimmer. Indeed it's a good idea to set yourself up well first thing in the morning. Skip breakfast and all that will happen is that you will find yourself wanting a snack mid-morning. So be like Julia and eat heartily and sensibly at breakfast time, and you just might find yourself edging a bit closer to that big-screen-friendly figure of hers. Here are some ideas for a healthy, hearty, slimming breakfast:

BREAKFAST 1

25g porridge oats with sweetener and skimmed milk (or, if you prefer the Scottish way, a little salt)
100g melon with a little chopped stem ginger
25g lean ham with 1 small crispbread

BREAKFAST 2

Sandwich of 2 slices wholemeal bread and 25g skinless cooked chicken
100g strawberries whizzed with 150ml fat-free plain yogurt
Small cup of drinking chocolate made with skimmed milk

BREAKFAST 3

50g grilled very lean bacon
2 grilled tomatoes
50g grilled mushrooms (sprayed with a little olive oil)
1 slice toast with 1 teaspoon low-fat spread
1 large apple

BREAKFAST 4

50g kipper fillets, grilled or cooked in a little water

1 slice wholemeal bread

1 small banana

Small low-fat yogurt

BREAKFAST 5

½ grapefruit with a little sweetener (if desired) and chopped mint

1-egg herb omelette served with 1 roasted pepper and

1 roasted tomato

1 slice toast with 1 small teaspoon low-fat spread and Marmite

BREAKFAST 6

1 large orange

Small can low-calorie baked beans and 50g grilled mushrooms on 25g wholemeal bread (no spread)

1 low-fat fruit yogurt

BREAKFAST 7

25g wholewheat cereal with skimmed milk

75g smoked haddock, cooked in a little skimmed milk and topped with 1 small poached egg

125g grapes

FAMOUS PEOPLE DON'T GET FAT

Kylie Minogue keeps that world-famous bum in trim for the hotpants by a combination of rollerblading, kick-boxing and yoga.

Gaby Roslin

A WHEAT-FREE regime is Gaby Roslin's key to keeping her figure TV-friendly. This is not as easy as it might sound – you'll find wheat or wheat flour in bread, biscuits, pasta, noodles, some cereals – the list goes on. But it can be a very effective way of keeping in trim, if only because a lot of foods containing wheat tend to have high sugar and fat contents too – just think of all those cakes and biscuits made with wheat flour.

In addition, some people have an intolerance or allergy to wheat, which stops them from absorbing food in the correct way. If you think this might apply to you, do seek professional advice.

You can buy wheat-free or gluten-free breads at health food shops and other specialist retailers (see page 302), but for the dieter eager to get started here are a few tasty recipes that work well in a wheat-free regime.

Slimmer's Lentil Soup

(Serves 4)

This is an excellent soup for a wheat-free diet because the lentils contain vitamin E, which you might be missing by avoiding products containing wheat.

175g lentils, washed and drained
2 teaspoons vegetable oil
2 carrots, chopped
2 medium onions, chopped
3 stalks celery, chopped
1 can tomatoes
2 garlic cloves, finely chopped
1.7 litres vegetable stock
1 teaspoon oregano, chopped
salt and pepper

Fry the carrots, onions and celery until slightly brown. Stir in the lentils, tomatoes and garlic, then add the stock. Bring to the boil, cover and simmer for about 1 hour. Add salt, pepper and oregano to taste, and serve.

Spicy Prawn Hotpot

(Serves 4)

225g raw prawns
2 cans tomatoes
1 teaspoon vegetable oil
2 shallots, sliced
½ teaspoon coriander seeds
½ teaspoon cumin seeds
½ teaspoon ground ginger
1 teaspoon turmeric powder
½ teaspoon chilli powder
salt and freshly ground black pepper

Fry the shallots in the oil until soft and golden. Add the coriander and cumin seeds, ginger and turmeric, and cook for about 1 minute. Add the prawns and tomatoes and stir well. Simmer for about 15 minutes so that the liquid thickens. Add the remaining prawns and simmer until pink and cooked. Season and serve with plain brown rice.

Cinnamony Baked Apples

(Serves 4)

4 large Bramley apples, cored

2 tablespoon raisins

2 tablespoons walnuts, chopped

1 teaspoon cinnamon

1 teaspoon low-calorie sweetener

Pre-heat the oven to 190°C/gas mark 5. When coring the apples, try not to cut all the way through to the bottom. Arrange them in a baking tray. Combine the raisins, walnuts, cinnamon and sweetener. Stuff each apple with the mixture. Bake for about 45 minutes until tender but not collapsing. You might like to baste the apples occasionally with their juice mixed with a little water.

Claudia Schiffer

BEAUTIFUL CLAUDIA Schiffer is one of the most glamorous and best-known models in the world, the envy of women everywhere. Claudia keeps her million-dollar shape by a strict dieting regime. Before noon she eats nothing but fruit. Her main meal tends to be at lunchtime, and in the evening she sticks to a very light meal of steamed vegetables.

It is a very good tip not to eat too heavily before you go to bed, as you don't burn up as many calories when you are asleep as you do when you're awake and moving around.

Here are a few ideas for some fruit breakfasts and mid-morning snacks that you can try in order to emulate Claudia's diet, and also some ways of making those evening steamed vegetables a bit more interesting:

Wild Fruit Salad

(Serves 1)
50g strawberries
a handful of mixed raspberries, blackberries and blueberries

Purée the strawberries, combine with the remaining fruit and serve.

Melon Surprise

(Serves 1)
½ melon (of any variety)
50g raspberries
50g seedless black grapes
juice of ½ orange

Remove the seeds from the centre of the melon. Fill with the raspberries and grapes, sprinkle with the orange juice and serve.

Baked Banana

(Serves 1)

This is one of the most satisfying things you can eat on a cold winter morning. Simply place a banana on a baking tray, pop it into an oven heated to 180°C/gas mark 4 and bake for about 15 minutes. When the skin has gone black, simply cut along the length of the banana and eat from the skin with a spoon. Careful – it's hot!

Toasted Pineapple

(Serves 1)

If you grill a skinned slice of pineapple under a grill, the natural sugars will caramelise and you'll be left with something quite delicious. Eat it on its own, or flavour it further with a drop of fresh orange or lemon juice, and maybe a sprinkling of mint or basil.

Steamed Vegetables

You can steam almost any vegetable. If you don't have a steamer, use a colander on top of a saucepan of boiling water and put a saucepan lid over the top. Steaming is a brilliant way of cooking vegetables, because:

- You don't need to use any extra fat.
- The vegetables retain many of the nutrients that might otherwise be removed by boiling.
- The natural taste of the vegetables is preserved, so it's a great cooking method for the foodie as well as the dieter.

Once you've steamed your vegetables, try flavouring them with low-calorie condiments. Soy sauce, oyster sauce, lemon juice and fresh herbs are all great ways of doing this – experiment and you'll find plenty of other things that also work well. Meanwhile, here are a couple of ideas to get your taste buds going:

Steamed Bok Choi with Oyster Sauce

(Serves 1)

2 young bok choi

2 tablespoons oyster sauce

Tabasco sauce

Steam the bok choi until they are cooked but retain some bite. Meanwhile, heat the oyster sauce in a saucepan with a couple of drops of Tabasco sauce (or more if you like a bit more heat). Spoon the sauce over the cooked bok choi and serve.

Steamed Broccoli with Sunflower Seeds

(Serves 1)

1 head of broccoli

1 tablespoon sunflower seeds

soy sauce (optional)

Peel the main stalk of the broccoli, cut into batons and steam with the florets until it is all nicely cooked. Chop the cooked broccoli roughly, mix it up with the sunflower seeds and a splash of soy sauce, if you fancy it, and serve.

Jane Seymour

THIS STAR of the silver screen admits to having an incredibly sweet tooth. If you are like Jane, then don't despair! You can't gorge on chocolate and sweets, but it doesn't mean you have to abandon your love of sweet things altogether. Jane enjoys the delicious, energy-boosting natural sugars in fruit by snacking on frozen fruit bars. You can make these yourself very easily. Buy some ice-lolly moulds from a kitchen shop, and let your imagination run riot.

You can either juice your own fruit or buy freshly squeezed, unsweetened juice from the supermarket. And don't just stop at boring old oranges – you can make frozen fruit bars from pineapple, grapefruit, strawberries, raspberries, apple (try adding a bit of cinnamon – delicious). The list is almost endless. All you need is a good-quality electric juicer, which you can use to produce all sorts of other tasty juices and smoothies (see pages 112-13 and 161).

Alicia Silverstone

LIKE DREW Barrymore, Alicia Silverstone follows a vegan diet in order to lose weight – no meat or fish products, and that includes milk and eggs. Followed sensibly, it can be a brilliant way of losing weight, so here are a few more recipes to get you started on your vegan diet plan:

Lentil Salad

(Serves 1)

125g lentils

4 pickled onions

2 medium tomatoes, peeled, seeded and diced

1 stick celery

1 lemon

1 fat garlic clove, crushed

1 tablespoon olive oil

1 teaspoon lemon juice

freshly ground black pepper

Wash the lentils carefully and cook them according to the instructions on the packet. When soft and most of the water has evaporated, purée them in a blender. Add the crushed garlic according to taste and season well with olive oil, lemon juice and plenty of black pepper. Mix into it slices of pickled onion and the tomatoes. Surround with curled celery and lemon quarters.

Squash and Bean Soup

(Serves 6)

1 butternut squash
225g dried white beans
1 medium onion, roughly chopped
2 garlic cloves, roughly chopped
1.7 litres vegetable stock
1½ tsp mixed dried herbs
1 bay leaf
450 ml skimmed milk
salt and freshly ground black pepper
½ teaspoon paprika
chopped parsley to garnish

Soak the beans overnight in cold water. Drain them and place in a large saucepan. Add the onion and garlic to the pan with 1.1 litres of the stock, 1 teaspoon of the dried herbs and the bay leaf. Bring to the boil then reduce the heat. Cover and simmer for about 1½ hours until the beans are tender.

Peel the squash and discard the seeds and membrane. Finely dice the flesh and simmer in the reserved stock and herbs for 15 minutes until tender.

Allow to cool, them remove the bay leaf from the beans, add the squash, milk and stock mixture and purée in a liquidiser until smooth.

Return to the pan and reheat gently. Season to taste, sprinkle paprika in the centre of each serving and garnish with the chopped parsley.

Summer Croustade

This is a slightly more complicated dish for a special occasion. Its success depends on achieving a crisp golden base and the very careful cooking and fresh appearance of the vegetables.

CROUSTADE

Medium-sized stale white loaf cut into 10cm x 12cm squares
Olive oil to brush the bread
2 garlic cloves, crushed with salt

FILLING

Summer vegetables (such as peas, broad beans, baby carrots, new potatoes, tiny beetroots or whatever you fancy)
chives or finely chopped mixed fresh herbs
French dressing

Add the garlic to the oil and brush on to one side of the bread squares. Oil a fireproof dish generously and arrange the squares in it, overlapping slightly, then fit a smaller tin inside the lined one to keep the bread in place, and bake in a moderate oven for about 30 minutes or until it is golden brown. Cool and turn out very carefully.

Meanwhile, prepare and cook all the vegetables separately and marinade them in the French dressing for about 1 hour.

To serve, lay the croustade on a flat dish, drain the vegetables from the marinade and arrange them attractively. Sprinkle on the chives or chopped herbs.

FAMOUS PEOPLE DON'T GET FAT

TV presenter *Amanda Lamb* always travels with a stash of supplements, so wherever her work takes her, she always has multivitamins to hand in case her schedule has her skipping meals.

Britney Spears

YEARS OF dancing has given pop sensation Britney Spears an impressive physique, proving that getting down on the dance floor can be one of the most effective ways to lose weight, keep fit and look fantastic.

But of course she watches what she eats too. Like Angelina Jolie and others, Britney's slimming secret is to eat five small meals a day. She avoids refined sugars and complex carbohydrates (bread, pasta and the like, which break down into natural sugar), avoids any carbohydrates later in the day, keeps her protein levels up and never eats after 8 pm (going to bed with a full stomach is a sure-fire way to pile on weight).

Here are some eating plans to get you on your way to a pop-star figure:

MENU 1

7 AM

2-egg omelette

½ slice wholemeal toast with low-fat spread

1 teaspoon marmalade

10 AM

50g cheese

1 apple

1 PM

Grilled chicken breast

Large mixed salad

Strawberries and 1 tablespoon low-fat crème fraîche

4 PM

Small bunch of grapes

7 PM

Cutlet of grilled salmon

1 tablespoon low-fat lemon mayonnaise

175g broccoli

175g fruit jelly

MENU 2

7 AM

50g grilled lean bacon

2 grilled tomatoes

10 AM

1 banana

1 PM

125g grilled lean fillet steak

125g mushrooms, cooked in a little oil, and 50g sugar snap peas

Stewed prunes

4 PM

1 small scone with low-fat spread and honey

7 PM

Stir-fry of sliced peppers, spring onions and bean sprouts topped with 125g prawns

2 slices fresh pineapple

Posh Spice *Victoria Beckham* is said to do 200 stomach crunches with husband David before they go to bed every night. And despite controversy about her weight, she claims to be a big eater, eating three solid meals a day – but always going for the healthier option. And maybe running around after Brooklyn, Romeo and Cruz helps keep her in trim too!

Martine McCutcheon loses weight by following the wacky 'blood group diet', which prescribes a different eating regime according to your blood group. Why not read *The Eat Right Diet* by Dr Peter D'Amono to see if there really is something in it?

MENU 3

7 AM

50g Cheddar cheese on ½ slice wholemeal bread

1 orange

10 AM

125g fresh fruit salad

1 PM

Grilled fillet of plaice with asparagus and courgettes

1 large slice melon

4 PM

2 sticks celery and 75g cottage cheese

7 PM

Grilled pork chop with apple sauce, steamed cabbage and steamed leeks

Banana custard

MENU 4

7 AM

2 low-fat sausages

Small can tomatoes, heated

1 pear

10 AM

Small pancake with strawberries

1 PM

125g roast chicken without skin

175g ratatouille (see page 97)

Fruit salad

4 PM

50g Parma ham and 2 fresh figs

7 PM

175g grilled breast of duck with orange sauce, large mixed salad and 2 very small new potatoes

MENU 5

7 AM

1 poached egg, creamed mushrooms and 1 grilled tomato

10 AM

1 slice wholemeal bread and Marmite

1 PM

1 small portion beef casserole served with steamed cabbage and cauliflower
6 dates

4 PM

1 pear with watercress and celery salad

7 PM

175g steamed monkfish with steamed leeks and wilted spinach
Rhubarb with sweetener and 2 tablespoons single cream

Catherine Zeta-Jones

FROM THE backwaters of Wales to the Hollywood A-list, Catherine Zeta-Jones has the celebrity career, celebrity husband and celebrity looks that so many people dream of. But it hasn't all been plain sailing. Catherine is as subject to the ups and downs of her weight as anyone. After the birth of her first child, she found that her weight was up by 19kg – and with only three months till her wedding to Michael Douglas.

How did she lose it? The way we all do – diet and exercise.

For her high-profile role in the Hollywood blockbuster *The Mask of Zorro*, Catherine took up fencing – a perfect way of toning her chest, upper arms and shoulders.

But if that sounds a bit too strenuous, you could try losing weight the Catherine Zeta-Jones way – by following a very low-carbohydrate dieting plan. The idea is that for the first two weeks you stick to protein-rich food, limiting your carbohydrate as far as possible. The great thing about diets like this is that you don't have to keep depriving yourself – as long as you are eating the right kind of food, you really don't have to go hungry. But do remember that a diet of this kind is not recommended for people who are not overweight – it's an intensive weight-loss programme that can cause you to burn muscle tissue if you are not careful.

Here are five high-protein, low-carbohydrate meals which will get you started on this regime. If you want to follow low-carb diets in more detail, the most famous ones, used by many celebrities around the world, are the Atkins and Zone diets. (See page 332 for more on these.)

You can drink as much decaffeinated coffee or tea, herbal teas, sparkling mineral water or soda water as you like. Mayonnaise should be home-made if possible with pure olive oil, fresh eggs and no sugar.

MENU I

BREAKFAST

20ml tomato juice
Eggs scrambled with butter
I rasher of streaky bacon

LUNCH

Steamed cauliflower, sprinkled with 50g Gruyere cheese and grilled
Small tossed salad

DINNER

Prawn cocktail
Roast chicken
2 large grilled mushrooms
50g spinach

DAY 2

BREAKFAST

Smoked salmon with 30g cream cheese on 12 slices cucumber

LUNCH

Grilled steak with garlic
60g grilled tomatoes
Green salad tossed with olive oil and a squeeze of lemon juice

DINNER

Caesar salad (no croutons)
Lightly griddled tuna steak with home-made mayonnaise
6 spears asparagus
60g broccoli

DAY 3

BREAKFAST

Bacon and 60g toasted cheese

30g grilled tomatoes

LUNCH

2 lamb cutlets

80g cabbage

30g peas

DINNER

Consommé

1 pancake (made with eggs and soya flour) stuffed with crab and mayonnaise

50g steamed French beans

Sugar-free jelly

DAY 4

BREAKFAST

Fried egg and bacon

LUNCH

1 large grilled pork chop

60g boiled swede mashed with butter

100g spinach

DINNER

Raw mushrooms and crispy bacon dressed with olive oil and lemon juice

Sea bass

Large tossed salad of lettuce, cucumber and radish

Sugar-free jelly with 30ml single cream

DAY 5

BREAKFAST

Grilled ham and poached egg

LUNCH

Cold chicken

Salad of lettuce, 4 rings green pepper, 4 slices cucumber

Home-made mayonnaise

DINNER

Prawns in garlic sauce

Roast leg of lamb with natural meat juices for gravy

80g spring greens

FAMOUS PEOPLE DON'T GET FAT

Dannii Minogue always takes the stairs – even when there's an elevator – in order to keep those leg muscles working and in trim.

Appendix

High-protein, Low-carbohydrate Diets

THESE ARE very popular, especially in America, where countless Hollywood stars have specially designed meals delivered to them on the set of their latest movie or TV show! We can't all afford that little luxury, but if you want to read more about these highly effective, very widely used diets, then the most popular are Dr Barry Sears's Zone Diet and the Atkins Diet devised by Dr Robert Atkins.

THE ZONE DIET

RECOMMENDED READING

The Zone Dr Barry Sears
(HarperCollins, 1996, ISBN 0060987162)

Mastering the Zone Dr Barry Sears
(HarperCollins, 1998, ISBN 0060929030)
Further information: www.drsears.com
www.zoneperfect.com

THE ATKINS DIET

RECOMMENDED READING

Dr Atkins' New Diet Revolution
Dr Robert Atkins
(Vermilion, 2003, ISBN 0091889480)

Dr Atkins' Quick and Easy New Diet Cookbook
Dr Robert Atkins
(Pocket Books, 2003, ISBN 0743462416)
Further information: www.atkinscenter.com

Organic Food

Many celebrities insist that the food they consume should be organic, and this is something the keen dieter would do very well to take on board, for a number of reasons. The most obvious is that the health benefits of organic food are beyond question. It is produced in a far more satisfactory manner, without the use of pesticides or other chemicals, and this alone should be reason enough to champion it. But additionally you will find that the more you concentrate on where your food comes from, the less you will be inclined to eat at random food you don't really want!

Most supermarkets now stock a reasonable range of organic food and drink, but you can investigate this field a great deal further by contacting the Soil Association at www.soilassociation.org

RECOMMENDED READING

The Joy of Organic Cookery Gilli Davies

(Metro Publishing, 2002, ISBN 1 84358 12 8)

Gluten-free Foods

As you will have read, a number of celebrity – and non-celebrity – slimmers periodically cut out wheat from their diet. Many people have to do this for medical reasons, and so there is a wide range of wheat- or gluten-free retailers available. Here are a few that you might find useful if you decide to opt for the wheat-free option:

GLUTEN FREE FOODS LTD,

Unit 270 Centennial Park, Centennial Avenue, Elstree,
Borehamwood, Hertfordshire WD6 3SS
Tel: 0208-953-4444
Fax: 0208-953-8285

RECOMMENDED READING

Everyday Gluten-Free Cooking Bette Hagman
(Metro Publishing, 2002, ISBN 1 84358 033 0)

Vegan Food

Drew Barrymore and Alicia Silverstone might be two of the most high-profile vegans in the world, but there are certainly plenty more. Veganism is a very successful way of slimming because you automatically cut out so many of the foodstuffs that are a slimmer's worst nightmare – no cream and butter for you! There are a number of resources and suppliers for vegans, which you can find from the following:

RECOMMENDED READING

The Joy of Vegan Cookery Amanda Grant
(Metro Publishing, 2003, ISBN 1 84358 023 3)
Further information: www.vegansociety.com

Ayurveda Medicine

The principles of Ayurveda yoga have been famously espoused as part of an integrated slimming regime by Geri Halliwell, but as we've already seen she's not the only celebrity to embrace its principles. Sting, Demi Moore and Nicole Kidman, to name but a few, have all been reported as fans of Ayurveda yoga. If you want to follow in their footsteps, contact:

www.practical-ayurveda.net
www.unifiedherbal.com

Tips for Eating Out

- Don't go to a restaurant feeling absolutely starving – it'll only encourage you to eat more. Instead, have a fat-free snack before you go out (apples are a good appetite suppressant).

- If you are ordering salad, ask for the dressing to be served on the side – that way you can control how much you use.

- Don't overdo it on the bread before the meal.

- Remember that nothing puts weight on like alcohol. If you really want to drink, limit it to a glass of wine with your meal.

Index of Recipes